Home Workouts That Work: Stay Fit Without the Gym

By Anthony Colasante

Table of Contents

Introduction

In today's fast-paced world, finding time to get to the gym can be a challenge. Whether it's due to a busy schedule, the inconvenience of commuting, or simply the desire for a more flexible workout routine, many people are turning to home workouts as a solution. The good news is that staying fit doesn't require expensive equipment or a gym membership. With the right approach, you can achieve your fitness goals from the comfort of your own home.

This book, *Home Workouts That Work: Stay Fit Without the Gym*, is designed to provide you with a comprehensive guide to effective home workouts that require little to no equipment. Whether you're a beginner or an advanced fitness enthusiast, you'll find routines and tips that fit your needs, helping you stay active, healthy, and motivated—all without leaving your house.

Why Home Workouts Work

Home workouts are more than just a convenient alternative to the gym—they can be just as effective, if not more so, when done correctly. One of the key reasons home workouts work is their accessibility. You can exercise anytime, anywhere, without the need for special equipment or gym facilities. This flexibility makes it easier to maintain a consistent routine, which is crucial for achieving long-term fitness goals.

Moreover, home workouts allow for a personalized fitness experience. You can choose exercises that suit your fitness level, preferences, and goals, creating a routine that's tailored specifically to you. Whether you're focusing on strength, endurance, flexibility, or a combination of all three, home workouts can be adapted to meet your needs.

Another advantage is the ability to integrate workouts into your daily life. Instead of setting aside hours to commute and exercise at a gym, you can fit short, effective workouts into your schedule.

This not only saves time but also makes it easier to stick to a routine, as you can work out when it's most convenient for you.

Benefits of Exercising at Home

Exercising at home comes with numerous benefits, many of which go beyond physical fitness. Here are some key advantages:

1. Time Efficiency: Without the need to commute to a gym, you can save a significant amount of time. This makes it easier to incorporate workouts into your daily routine, even on the busiest days.
2. Cost Savings: Gym memberships, personal trainers, and specialized equipment can be expensive. Home workouts eliminate these costs, making fitness accessible to everyone.
3. Privacy and Comfort: Working out at home allows you to exercise in a comfortable and private environment. This can be especially beneficial for those who feel self-conscious at the gym or prefer to exercise alone.
4. Flexibility: Home workouts offer the flexibility to exercise whenever you want. Whether you're an early bird or a night owl, you can work out at a time that suits you best.
5. Customization: You have full control over your workout routine. You can choose exercises that you enjoy, adjust the intensity to match your fitness level, and create a schedule that fits your lifestyle.
6. Consistency: The convenience of home workouts makes it easier to maintain a consistent routine, which is essential for long-term success.

Overcoming Common Excuses

While the benefits of home workouts are clear, many people still struggle with making exercise a regular habit. Here are some common excuses and how to overcome them:

1. "I don't have enough time."
   - Solution: Home workouts can be as short as 10-15 minutes. Focus on high-intensity, efficient routines that maximize your time. Remember, consistency is more important than duration.
1. "I don't have any equipment."
   - Solution: Many effective workouts can be done using just your body weight. This book includes a variety of exercises that require little to no equipment, so you can get started with what you have.
1. "I don't know where to start."
   - Solution: This book is your guide. It provides structured workout plans for all fitness levels, so you can start with the basics and progress at your own pace.
1. "I get bored easily."
   - Solution: Variety is key to staying engaged. Mix up your routine with different types of workouts—strength training, cardio, flexibility exercises—to keep things interesting.
1. "I'm not motivated."
   -

      Solution: Set specific, achievable goals and track your progress. Celebrate small victories along the way, and remember why you started. Surround yourself with motivational resources, such as this book, to keep your spirits high.

By addressing these common challenges, you can remove the barriers that often prevent people from sticking to a workout routine. With the right mindset and approach, you'll find that home workouts are not just a temporary solution, but a sustainable way to achieve and maintain your fitness goals.

Chapter 1: Getting Started with Home Workouts

Embarking on a fitness journey from the comfort of your home can be both exciting and overwhelming. With so many exercises, routines, and tips out there, it's easy to feel lost, especially if you're just getting started. This chapter will guide you through the foundational steps to ensure that your home workout routine is effective, sustainable, and tailored to your unique needs.

Assessing Your Fitness Level

Before diving into a workout routine, it's crucial to assess your current fitness level. Understanding where you stand physically will help you choose the right exercises and set achievable goals. Here's how you can assess your fitness level:

1. **Cardiovascular Endurance:** Measure how long you can sustain a moderate-intensity activity like jogging, cycling, or brisk walking. Note how you feel during and after the activity—are you breathless, tired, or comfortable?
2. **Muscular Strength:** Test your strength with exercises like push-ups, squats, or planks. Record how many repetitions you can perform with good form before feeling fatigued.
3. **Flexibility:** Evaluate your flexibility with simple stretches like reaching for your toes or doing a forward bend. How far can you stretch without discomfort?
4. **Balance:** Try standing on one leg for as long as possible. Can you hold your balance for 30 seconds or more?
5. **Body Composition:** If possible, measure your body composition, including weight, body fat percentage, and muscle mass. While not essential, this can provide a baseline to track your progress.

Once you've assessed your fitness level, you can better tailor your workouts to your current abilities and gradually increase the intensity as you progress.

Setting Realistic Fitness Goals

Setting goals is a powerful way to stay motivated and track your progress. However, it's important to set goals that are realistic, specific, and achievable. Here's how to set effective fitness goals:

1. **Be Specific:** Instead of setting vague goals like "get fit" or "lose weight," be specific. For example, "I want to do 20 push-ups in a row" or "I want to lose 10 pounds in three months."
2. **Make Them Measurable:** Choose goals that you can measure. This could be the number of reps you can do, the distance you can run, or the amount of weight you can lift.
3. **Set a Time Frame:** Give yourself a deadline to achieve your goals. This helps create a sense of urgency and keeps you on track. For example, "I want to improve my flexibility enough to touch my toes within six weeks."
4. **Ensure They Are Achievable:** While it's great to aim high, your goals should be attainable given your current fitness level and lifestyle. Setting overly ambitious goals can lead to frustration and burnout.
5. **Be Realistic:** Consider your daily schedule, responsibilities, and other factors that might affect your ability to work out. Set goals that you can realistically incorporate into your life.
6. **Keep It Relevant:** Your goals should align with your overall fitness objectives, whether it's improving strength, endurance, flexibility, or weight management.

Remember to regularly review and adjust your goals as you progress. Celebrate your achievements, no matter how small, and use them as motivation to keep going.

Essential Equipment (And Alternatives You Already Have)

One of the best things about home workouts is that they often require little to no equipment. However, having some basic tools can enhance your workouts and add variety. Here's a list of essential equipment and alternatives you might already have at home:

1. **Resistance Bands:** These versatile tools are great for strength training and can be easily stored. They come in different resistance levels to match your fitness level.
   - **Alternative:** Use a pair of old tights or stockings for a similar effect.
1. **Dumbbells:** A set of dumbbells can be used for various exercises to build strength. If you're just starting, choose lighter weights and gradually increase as you get stronger.
   - **Alternative:** Use water bottles, canned goods, or bags filled with sand or rice.
1. **Yoga Mat:** A mat provides cushioning for floor exercises and yoga routines, making your workouts more comfortable.
   - **Alternative:** Use a towel or a blanket on a carpeted floor if you don't have a yoga mat.
1. **Stability Ball:** Great for core workouts, stability balls can add an extra challenge to exercises.
   -

Alternative: If you don't have a stability ball, you can use a firm pillow or cushion for some exercises.

1. **Jump Rope:** Jumping rope is an excellent cardio exercise that also improves coordination and agility.
   - **Alternative:** If you don't have a jump rope, you can mimic the movement or try high knees or jumping jacks.

1. **Chairs and Stairs:** Chairs can be used for exercises like tricep dips or step-ups, while stairs are perfect for cardio and lower body workouts.

   - **Alternative:** Use a sturdy table edge or a low wall for step-ups and other similar exercises.

You don't need to invest in expensive equipment to get a good workout at home. By using what you already have and getting creative with alternatives, you can still achieve a great workout.

Creating a Workout Space at Home

Creating a dedicated workout space at home can help you stay focused and motivated. It doesn't need to be a large area, but it should be a space where you feel comfortable and free to move. Here are some tips for setting up your workout space:

1. **Choose a Spot:** Find a spot in your home where you can exercise without interruptions. It could be a corner of your living room, bedroom, or even a garage or basement.
2. **Clear the Area:** Make sure the space is clear of clutter and obstacles. You'll need enough room to move freely, especially for exercises that require space, like jumping or stretching.
3. **Ensure Good Lighting:** A well-lit space can boost your mood and energy levels. Natural light is ideal,

but if that's not possible, make sure the area is well-lit with artificial light.

4. **Ventilation:** Ensure your workout space is well-ventilated. Fresh air can help keep you cool and energized during your workouts. If possible, open a window or use a fan.
5. **Keep Your Equipment Handy:** Store your workout equipment nearby so you can easily access it when needed. A basket or shelf can help keep things organized.
6. **Personalize Your Space:** Add personal touches to your workout space to make it more inviting. This could include motivational posters, a mirror, or a speaker for playing music.
7. **Safety First:** Make sure your workout space is safe. Ensure the floor is not slippery, there's adequate padding for floor exercises, and any equipment you use is in good condition.

By creating a dedicated workout space, you set the stage for success. It helps signal to your mind and body that it's time to focus on fitness, making it easier to stick to your routine.

With these foundational steps, you're well on your way to establishing a successful home workout routine. Remember, the key to success is starting where you are, setting achievable goals, and creating an environment that supports your fitness journey.

Chapter 2: Warm-Up and Cool-Down Routines

Warming up before exercise and cooling down afterward are essential components of any workout routine. These practices not only prepare your body for the physical demands of exercise but also aid in recovery, reducing the risk of injury and enhancing overall performance. This chapter will guide you through the importance of warming up and cooling down, along with effective techniques for each.

Importance of Warming Up and Cooling Down

Many people are tempted to skip the warm-up or cool-down, especially when time is limited. However, these phases are crucial for several reasons:

1. **Preparing the Body for Exercise:**
   - A proper warm-up gradually increases your heart rate, breathing, and blood flow to the muscles. This prepares your body for more intense activity by loosening the joints, warming up the muscles, and improving overall mobility. It also helps to mentally prepare you for the workout ahead, signaling to your body that it's time to focus.
1. **Preventing Injury:**
   - Warming up helps to prevent injuries by increasing the elasticity of the muscles and improving joint range of motion. This reduces the risk of strains, sprains, and other injuries that can occur when muscles are cold and tight. Similarly, cooling down helps to gradually reduce your heart rate and stretch out tight muscles, which can prevent cramps and stiffness.
1. **Enhancing Performance:**

○

A good warm-up can enhance your performance by improving muscle efficiency and coordination. When your body is properly prepared, you can exercise more effectively, with better form and less fatigue.

1. **Aiding in Recovery:**
   ○

   Cooling down after exercise helps to prevent blood from pooling in the muscles, which can cause dizziness or fainting. It also aids in the removal of metabolic waste products, such as lactic acid, which can contribute to muscle soreness. Cooling down also provides an opportunity to relax and mentally unwind after a workout.

Incorporating both warm-up and cool-down routines into your workouts is a simple yet effective way to enhance your exercise experience and ensure long-term success.

Dynamic Stretching for a Safe Start

Dynamic stretching is a form of stretching that involves active movements that take your muscles and joints through their full range of motion. Unlike static stretching, where you hold a stretch for a period of time, dynamic stretching is more fluid and helps to increase blood flow, improve flexibility, and prepare your muscles for the movements you'll perform during your workout. Here are some key dynamic stretches to include in your warm-up:

1. **Leg Swings:**
   ○

   Stand next to a wall or a sturdy surface for support. Swing one leg forward and backward in a controlled motion, gradually increasing the range of motion. Repeat on the other leg. This stretch targets your hip flexors, hamstrings, and glutes.

1. **Arm Circles:**

   - Stand with your feet shoulder-width apart and extend your arms out to the sides. Make small circles with your arms, gradually increasing the size of the circles. Reverse the direction after a few rotations. This movement warms up the shoulders and improves mobility.

1. **Lunges with a Twist:**

   - Step forward into a lunge position, keeping your back straight and your knee aligned over your ankle. As you lunge, twist your torso towards the leading leg. Return to the starting position and repeat on the other side. This dynamic stretch engages the hips, quads, hamstrings, and core.

1. **High Knees:**

   - Stand with your feet hip-width apart and lift one knee towards your chest, then quickly switch to the other knee in a marching or jogging motion. This exercise warms up the legs, core, and cardiovascular system.

1. **Hip Circles:**

   - Stand with your feet shoulder-width apart and place your hands on your hips. Slowly rotate your hips in a circular motion, first in one direction, then in the other. This movement helps to loosen the hip joints and lower back.

1. **Torso Twists:**

   -

   Stand with your feet shoulder-width apart and arms extended in front of you. Twist your torso from side to side, allowing your arms to follow the movement. This stretch targets the obliques and warms up the spine.

Perform each of these dynamic stretches for 30 seconds to one minute, ensuring that your movements are controlled and not forced. This will effectively prepare your body for the workout ahead, reducing the risk of injury and improving your performance.

Post-Workout Stretching: Relax and Recover

After a workout, your muscles are warm and pliable, making it the perfect time for static stretching. Static stretching involves holding a stretch for a longer period (typically 15-30 seconds) to lengthen the muscles, increase flexibility, and promote relaxation. Here are some essential stretches to include in your cool-down routine:

1. **Hamstring Stretch:**
   - Sit on the floor with one leg extended straight and the other bent, with the sole of your foot against the inner thigh of your extended leg. Reach towards your toes, keeping your back straight. Hold the stretch, then switch legs. This stretch targets the hamstrings and lower back.
1. **Quad Stretch:**
   - Stand on one leg, holding onto a wall or chair for balance if needed. Bend the other knee and bring your heel towards your glutes, holding your ankle with your hand. Keep your knees close together and push your hips forward slightly to deepen the stretch. Switch legs after holding the stretch. This targets the quadriceps and hip flexors.
1. **Chest Stretch:**
   - Stand with your feet shoulder-width apart and clasp your hands behind your back. Straighten your arms

and lift them slightly while opening your chest and pulling your shoulders back. This stretch opens up the chest and shoulders, which can become tight from upper body exercises.

1. **Child's Pose:**
   -

   Kneel on the floor and sit back on your heels. Extend your arms forward and lower your torso towards the floor, resting your forehead on the ground. This stretch relaxes the lower back, shoulders, and arms while promoting deep breathing.

1. **Calf Stretch:**
   -

   Stand facing a wall, placing your hands on the wall at shoulder height. Step one foot back and press the heel into the ground while keeping the leg straight. Lean into the wall to deepen the stretch. Hold, then switch legs. This stretch targets the calf muscles, which can become tight after lower body exercises.

1. **Hip Flexor Stretch:**
   -

   Kneel on one knee with the other foot in front, forming a 90-degree angle with both legs. Push your hips forward, keeping your back straight, until you feel a stretch in the hip flexor of the back leg. Hold, then switch sides. This stretch targets the hip flexors and can help alleviate tightness from sitting or running.

1. **Lower Back Stretch:**
   -

   Lie on your back and bring both knees towards your chest, hugging them with your arms. Gently rock from side to side to massage the lower back. This stretch relaxes the lower back and helps to release tension.

Hold each stretch for at least 15-30 seconds, breathing deeply and allowing your muscles to relax. Avoid bouncing or forcing the stretch—focus on gently lengthening the muscles and enjoying the post-workout relaxation. Incorporating these static stretches into your cool-down routine will help improve flexibility, reduce muscle soreness, and promote a sense of well-being after your workout.

By prioritizing warm-up and cool-down routines, you're not only protecting yourself from injury but also enhancing the overall effectiveness of your workouts. These routines set the tone for your exercise session and help you transition smoothly into recovery, making them indispensable components of your fitness regimen.

Chapter 3: Bodyweight Exercises for Beginners

Bodyweight exercises are a fantastic way to build strength, improve flexibility, and enhance overall fitness without the need for any equipment. For beginners, these exercises provide a solid foundation, allowing you to master basic movements, build confidence, and progressively challenge your body. This chapter will introduce you to the world of bodyweight training, guide you through a beginner-friendly workout routine, and offer tips on how to track your progress.

Introduction to Bodyweight Training

Bodyweight training uses your own body as resistance to build strength, endurance, and mobility. It's one of the most versatile and accessible forms of exercise, as it can be done anywhere, at any time, without the need for equipment. Here are some key benefits of bodyweight training:

1. **Accessibility:** Since no equipment is required, bodyweight exercises can be performed in any environment—whether you're at home, traveling, or even outdoors.
2. **Scalability:** Bodyweight exercises can be easily modified to suit your fitness level. As a beginner, you can start with the basics and gradually increase the intensity by adjusting the number of repetitions, sets, or by adding variations to the exercises.
3. **Functional Fitness:** Bodyweight exercises often mimic movements you perform in daily life, helping you improve functional strength and mobility. This can make everyday tasks easier and reduce the risk of injury.
4. **Improved Coordination and Balance:** Many bodyweight exercises engage multiple muscle groups and require a higher degree of coordination and balance, leading to better overall body control.

5. **Efficient Workouts:** Bodyweight exercises often engage multiple muscle groups simultaneously, allowing you to get a full-body workout in a short amount of time.

As you embark on your bodyweight training journey, focus on mastering the fundamental movements. These exercises will form the basis of your routine and help you build a strong foundation.

Full-Body Beginner Workout Routine

This beginner workout routine is designed to target all major muscle groups, helping you build strength and endurance while improving your overall fitness. The routine can be completed in 20-30 minutes and requires no equipment. Perform this workout 2-3 times per week, allowing at least one day of rest between sessions.

Warm-Up (5 Minutes):

- **Jumping Jacks:** 1 minute
- **Arm Circles:** 30 seconds each direction
- **Leg Swings:** 30 seconds per leg
- **Torso Twists:** 1 minute

Workout:

1. **Squats:**
   - **Reps:** 10-15
   - **Sets:** 2-3
   -

Instructions: Stand with your feet shoulder-width apart, toes slightly turned out. Lower your body as if sitting back into a chair, keeping your chest up and knees tracking over your toes. Push through your heels to return to the starting position.

1. **Push-Ups:**
   - **Reps:** 8-12
   - **Sets:** 2-3
   - **Instructions:** Begin in a plank position with your hands slightly wider than shoulder-width apart. Lower your body until your chest is just above the floor, then push back up to the starting position. Modify by dropping to your knees if needed.
1. **Glute Bridges:**
   - **Reps:** 12-15
   - **Sets:** 2-3
   - **Instructions:** Lie on your back with your knees bent and feet flat on the floor, hip-width apart. Lift your hips towards the ceiling, squeezing your glutes at the top. Lower your hips back down without touching the floor, and repeat.
1. **Plank:**
   - **Time:** 20-30 seconds
   - **Sets:** 2-3
   - **Instructions:** Begin in a forearm plank position with your body in a straight line from head to heels. Engage your core, avoiding sagging or arching your back. Hold for the allotted time.

1. **Lunges:**
   -
   Reps: 8-12 per leg
   -
   Sets: 2-3
   -
   Instructions: Stand with your feet together. Step forward with one leg and lower your body until both knees are bent at 90 degrees. Push through the front heel to return to the starting position. Repeat on the other leg.
1. **Bird-Dog:**
   -
   Reps: 10-12 per side
   -
   Sets: 2-3
   -

   Instructions: Begin on your hands and knees in a tabletop position. Extend your right arm forward and left leg back, keeping your core engaged. Return to the starting position and repeat on the other side.

Cool-Down (5 Minutes):

-
Hamstring Stretch: 30 seconds per leg
-
Quad Stretch: 30 seconds per leg
-
Chest Stretch: 30 seconds
-

Child's Pose: 1 minute

This routine covers the essential movements that will help you build a strong foundation. As you become more comfortable with these exercises, you can gradually increase the number of sets or repetitions, or try more challenging variations.

Progress Tracking: Seeing Your Improvements

Tracking your progress is an essential part of any fitness journey. It allows you to see how far you've come, stay motivated, and make necessary adjustments to your routine. Here's how to effectively track your progress:

1. **Keep a Workout Journal:**
   - Record your workouts, including the exercises you performed, the number of sets and repetitions, and how you felt during and after the workout. This will help you track your improvements over time and identify any patterns.
1. **Take Measurements:**
   - In addition to tracking your strength and endurance, consider taking body measurements, such as waist, hips, and chest, to monitor changes in your body composition. This can be especially motivating if weight loss or muscle gain is one of your goals.
1. **Set Short-Term Goals:**
   - Break down your long-term goals into smaller, achievable milestones. For example, aim to increase the number of push-ups you can do by 2-3 each week. Celebrate these small victories to keep your motivation high.
1. **Use Progress Photos:**
   - Take photos of yourself at regular intervals, such as every 4-6 weeks. Seeing the physical changes in your body can be incredibly motivating, especially

if you're not noticing immediate changes on the scale.

1. **Listen to Your Body:**
   -
   Pay attention to how your body feels as you progress. Are you finding the exercises easier? Do you have more energy throughout the day? Are you recovering faster? These are all signs of improvement.

1. **Reassess Your Fitness Level:**
   -
   Every 4-6 weeks, reassess your fitness level using the same methods you used in Chapter 1. Compare your results to your initial assessment to see how far you've come.

1. **Adjust Your Routine:**
   -

   As you progress, your body will adapt to the exercises, and you may need to adjust your routine to continue seeing improvements. Increase the intensity by adding more repetitions, sets, or trying more advanced variations of the exercises.

By consistently tracking your progress, you'll gain valuable insights into your fitness journey and be better equipped to make informed decisions about your workout routine. Remember, progress takes time, so be patient with yourself and celebrate every achievement, no matter how small.

With this foundation in bodyweight exercises, you're well on your way to building strength, improving your fitness, and setting the stage for more advanced workouts in the future. Remember, the key to success is consistency—stick with your routine, track your progress, and keep challenging yourself as you grow stronger.

Chapter 4: Intermediate Home Workout Routines

Once you've established a solid foundation with beginner bodyweight exercises, it's time to take your workouts to the next level. This chapter focuses on intermediate home workout routines that introduce more challenging bodyweight exercises, incorporate cardio and plyometrics to increase intensity, and provide a comprehensive full-body workout plan designed to build strength, endurance, and overall fitness.

Stepping Up: Intermediate Bodyweight Exercises

As you progress in your fitness journey, it's important to continue challenging your muscles with more advanced exercises. Intermediate bodyweight exercises build on the basics, offering variations that target your muscles in new ways and increase the difficulty. Here are some key intermediate exercises to incorporate into your routine:

1. **Pistol Squats:**
   - **Instructions:** Stand on one leg with the other leg extended in front of you. Lower your body into a squat, keeping your extended leg off the ground. Push through your heel to return to the starting position. This exercise targets the quads, glutes, and core, while also improving balance and stability.
1. **Decline Push-Ups:**
   - **Instructions:** Place your feet on an elevated surface (such as a bench or chair) and perform a push-up. This variation increases the difficulty by placing more emphasis on the upper chest and shoulders.
1. **Bulgarian Split Squats:**
   -

Instructions: Stand a few feet in front of a bench or chair, with one foot resting on the surface behind you. Lower your body into a lunge, keeping your front knee aligned with your ankle. Push through your front heel to return to the starting position. This exercise targets the quads, glutes, and hamstrings, while also improving balance.

1. **Diamond Push-Ups:**
   - **Instructions:** Position your hands close together under your chest, forming a diamond shape with your thumbs and index fingers. Lower your body into a push-up, keeping your elbows close to your sides. This variation targets the triceps and inner chest.

1. **Lateral Lunges:**
   - **Instructions:** Stand with your feet hip-width apart. Step to the side with one leg, lowering your body into a lunge while keeping the other leg straight. Push through your heel to return to the starting position and repeat on the other side. This exercise targets the inner thighs, glutes, and quads.

1. **Plank to Push-Up:**
   -

   Instructions: Start in a forearm plank position. Push up onto your hands, one hand at a time, until you're in a full plank position. Lower back down to the forearm plank. This exercise targets the core, shoulders, and chest, while also improving coordination and stability.

These intermediate exercises will help you continue to build strength and endurance, challenging your muscles in new ways and preparing you for even more advanced movements.

Adding Intensity: Cardio and Plyometrics

To further enhance your workouts and improve cardiovascular fitness, it's beneficial to incorporate cardio and plyometric exercises. Plyometrics, or jump training, involve explosive movements that increase power, speed, and agility. When combined with cardio exercises, they elevate your heart rate, burn calories, and boost overall fitness. Here are some key exercises to add intensity to your routine:

1. **Burpees:**
   - **Instructions:** Start in a standing position, then drop into a squat and place your hands on the floor. Jump your feet back into a plank position, perform a push-up, then jump your feet back to your hands and explosively jump into the air. This full-body exercise is excellent for cardio and strength.
1. **Jump Squats:**
   - **Instructions:** Perform a regular squat, but instead of standing up, explode into a jump, reaching your arms overhead. Land softly and immediately lower into the next squat. This plyometric exercise targets the quads, glutes, and calves, while also increasing heart rate.
1. **Mountain Climbers:**
   - **Instructions:** Start in a plank position. Quickly alternate bringing one knee towards your chest, then switching to the other, as if running in place. This exercise targets the core, shoulders, and legs, while providing a great cardio workout.
1. **High Knees:**
   - **Instructions:** Stand with your feet hip-width apart. Run in place, bringing your knees up towards your

chest as high as possible. Pump your arms as you move. This cardio exercise engages the core, legs, and improves coordination.

1. **Box Jumps:**
    - **Instructions:** Stand in front of a sturdy box or platform. Bend your knees and explode upwards, landing softly on the box with both feet. Step down and repeat. This plyometric exercise builds lower body power and explosiveness.

1. **Lateral Bounds:**
    -

        Instructions: Stand on one leg and leap sideways to land on the opposite leg, absorbing the impact with a slight bend in the knee. Repeat, bounding back and forth. This exercise improves lateral movement, balance, and leg strength.

Incorporating these high-intensity exercises into your routine will not only help you burn more calories but also improve your cardiovascular fitness and build explosive strength.

Intermediate Full-Body Workout Plan

This intermediate workout plan combines the advanced bodyweight exercises and plyometrics introduced earlier, creating a comprehensive full-body routine. Aim to perform this workout 3-4 times per week, with at least one rest day in between sessions.

Warm-Up (5-7 Minutes):

- **Jump Rope or High Knees:** 1-2 minutes
- **Leg Swings:** 30 seconds per leg
- **Arm Circles:** 30 seconds each direction

-

Torso Twists: 1 minute

Workout:

1. **Pistol Squats:**
   - **Reps:** 6-8 per leg
   - **Sets:** 3
   - **Instructions:** Perform the pistol squat as described earlier. Use a chair or wall for balance if needed.
1. **Decline Push-Ups:**
   - **Reps:** 10-12
   - **Sets:** 3
   - **Instructions:** Perform decline push-ups as described earlier. Focus on controlled movements and full range of motion.
1. **Bulgarian Split Squats:**
   - **Reps:** 10-12 per leg
   - **Sets:** 3
   - **Instructions:** Perform Bulgarian split squats as described earlier. Ensure your front knee stays aligned with your ankle.
1. **Burpees:**
   - **Reps:** 10-15
   - **Sets:** 3
   -

Instructions: Perform burpees as described earlier. Focus on maintaining a steady pace.

1. **Diamond Push-Ups:**
   - **Reps:** 8-10
   - **Sets:** 3
   - **Instructions:** Perform diamond push-ups as described earlier. Keep your core engaged and elbows close to your body.
1. **Jump Squats:**
   - **Reps:** 12-15
   - **Sets:** 3
   - **Instructions:** Perform jump squats as described earlier. Land softly and immediately transition into the next jump.
1. **Plank to Push-Up:**
   - **Reps:** 8-10
   - **Sets:** 3
   - **Instructions:** Perform plank to push-up as described earlier. Maintain a strong core throughout the movement.
1. **Mountain Climbers:**
   - **Time:** 30-45 seconds
   - **Sets:** 3
   -

Instructions: Perform mountain climbers as described earlier. Keep a steady pace and focus on core engagement.

Cool-Down (5 Minutes):

- **Hamstring Stretch:** 30 seconds per leg
- **Quad Stretch:** 30 seconds per leg
- **Chest Stretch:** 30 seconds
-

Child's Pose: 1 minute

This workout plan is designed to challenge your strength, endurance, and cardiovascular fitness. As you progress, you can further increase the intensity by adding more sets, repetitions, or reducing rest times between exercises.

By stepping up to these intermediate exercises and integrating cardio and plyometric movements, you're taking your home workouts to the next level. Remember to listen to your body, progress at your own pace, and continue challenging yourself as you build towards more advanced routines.

Chapter 5: Advanced Home Workout Challenges

As you continue to progress in your fitness journey, it's time to push your limits and take on more challenging exercises and routines. This chapter introduces advanced bodyweight techniques, explores the benefits of High-Intensity Interval Training (HIIT), and provides a comprehensive full-body workout routine designed to test your strength, endurance, and mental toughness.

Advanced Bodyweight Techniques

Advanced bodyweight exercises require greater strength, balance, and coordination. These movements not only challenge your muscles but also test your ability to control your body through complex motions. Here are some advanced bodyweight techniques to incorporate into your routine:

1. **One-Arm Push-Ups:**
   - **Instructions:** Begin in a standard push-up position, then place one hand behind your back. Lower your body slowly with the other hand until your chest nearly touches the floor. Push back up with control. This exercise targets the chest, triceps, shoulders, and core, while also requiring significant balance and stability.
1. **Handstand Push-Ups:**
   - **Instructions:** Kick up into a handstand against a wall for support. Lower your body by bending your elbows until your head nearly touches the floor, then push back up. This advanced movement primarily targets the shoulders and triceps, while also engaging the core and improving balance.
1. **L-Sit:**
   -

Instructions: Sit on the floor with your legs extended straight in front of you and your hands by your sides. Lift your body off the ground by pushing through your hands, keeping your legs straight and off the floor. Hold this position, engaging your core and hip flexors. The L-sit is a powerful core exercise that also builds strength in the shoulders and triceps.

1. **Plyometric Push-Ups:**
   - **Instructions:** Perform a push-up, but as you push up, explode off the ground with enough force to lift your hands off the floor. Clap your hands together before catching yourself and lowering back into the next push-up. This explosive movement builds power in the chest, triceps, and shoulders, while also engaging the core.

1. **Archer Pull-Ups:**
   - **Instructions:** Perform a pull-up, but as you pull your body up, shift most of your weight to one side, extending the opposite arm straight out to the side. Lower back down and repeat on the other side. Archer pull-ups are an advanced variation that targets the lats, biceps, and forearms, while also requiring significant core stability.

1. **Pistol Squat to Jump:**
   -

   Instructions: Perform a pistol squat as described in the intermediate section, but at the bottom of the movement, explode upwards into a jump, landing softly on the same leg. This exercise combines strength, balance, and explosive power, targeting the quads, glutes, and core.

These advanced techniques should only be attempted once you have mastered the foundational movements and have built the necessary strength and stability. Always prioritize form and control over speed to prevent injury.

High-Intensity Interval Training (HIIT) at Home

High-Intensity Interval Training (HIIT) is a powerful way to burn fat, build endurance, and improve cardiovascular fitness in a short amount of time. HIIT involves alternating between short bursts of intense exercise and brief periods of rest or low-intensity exercise. This training method keeps your heart rate elevated, maximizing calorie burn and boosting your metabolism. Here's how you can incorporate HIIT into your home workouts:

1. **Structure of a HIIT Workout:**
   - A typical HIIT workout consists of 20-40 seconds of high-intensity exercise followed by 10-20 seconds of rest. This cycle is repeated for a set number of rounds, usually lasting 15-30 minutes in total.
1. **Benefits of HIIT:**
   - **Efficiency:** HIIT workouts are time-efficient, allowing you to get a great workout in a short amount of time.
   - **Calorie Burn:** The intense bursts of exercise elevate your heart rate and increase calorie burn both during and after the workout.
   - **Improved Cardiovascular Health:** HIIT improves cardiovascular fitness by challenging your heart and lungs to work harder.
   -

Versatility: HIIT can be adapted to various exercises, making it easy to create new and challenging routines.

1. **Sample HIIT Exercises:**
    - **Burpees:** 30 seconds on, 15 seconds rest
    - **Mountain Climbers:** 30 seconds on, 15 seconds rest
    - **Jump Squats:** 30 seconds on, 15 seconds rest
    - **High Knees:** 30 seconds on, 15 seconds rest
    - **Push-Up to Plank:** 30 seconds on, 15 seconds rest
1. **HIIT Workout Plan:**
    - **Warm-Up:** 5 minutes of light cardio (e.g., jogging in place, jumping jacks)
    - **HIIT Circuit:** Perform each exercise for 30 seconds, followed by 15 seconds of rest. Complete the circuit 3-4 times with a 1-minute rest between rounds.
    - **Cool-Down:** 5 minutes of stretching and deep breathing

HIIT is highly effective, but it's also demanding. Listen to your body, and start with shorter intervals if needed, gradually increasing the intensity as your fitness improves.

Advanced Full-Body Workout Routine

This advanced workout routine combines the challenging bodyweight exercises and HIIT principles introduced earlier. Designed to test your limits, this routine targets all major muscle groups, building strength, endurance, and explosive power. Perform this workout 3 times per week, with at least one rest day between sessions.

Warm-Up (5-7 Minutes):

- **Jump Rope or High Knees:** 2 minutes
- **Leg Swings:** 30 seconds per leg
- **Arm Circles:** 30 seconds each direction

- **Torso Twists:** 1 minute

Workout:

1. **One-Arm Push-Ups:**
   - **Reps:** 4-6 per arm
   - **Sets:** 3
   - **Instructions:** Perform one-arm push-ups as described earlier. Focus on maintaining control and balance throughout the movement.
1. **Pistol Squat to Jump:**
   - **Reps:** 6-8 per leg
   - **Sets:** 3
   - **Instructions:** Perform pistol squats to jump as described earlier. Land softly and immediately transition into the next rep.
1. **L-Sit:**
   -

Time: 20-30 seconds

o

Sets: 3

o

Instructions: Hold the L-sit position as described earlier. Focus on engaging your core and maintaining straight legs.

1. **Handstand Push-Ups:**

   o

   Reps: 4-6

   o

   Sets: 3

   o

   Instructions: Perform handstand push-ups as described earlier. Use a wall for support and focus on controlled movements.

1. **Burpees:**

   o

   Reps: 10-12

   o

   Sets: 3

   o

   Instructions: Perform burpees as described earlier. Maintain a steady pace and focus on form.

1. **Archer Pull-Ups:**

   o

   Reps: 6-8 per side

   o

   Sets: 3

   o

   Instructions: Perform archer pull-ups as described earlier. Alternate sides with each rep, ensuring full range of motion.

1. **Plyometric Push-Ups:**

   o

   Reps: 8-10

   o

Sets: 3

o

Instructions: Perform plyometric push-ups as described earlier. Explode off the ground with each rep, clapping your hands together at the top.

1. **HIIT Circuit:**

o

Structure: 30 seconds on, 15 seconds rest

o

Exercises: Jump Squats, Mountain Climbers, High Knees, Push-Up to Plank

o

Rounds: 3-4

o

Rest: 1 minute between rounds

Cool-Down (5 Minutes):

-

Hamstring Stretch: 30 seconds per leg

-

Quad Stretch: 30 seconds per leg

-

Chest Stretch: 30 seconds

-

Child's Pose: 1 minute

This advanced routine is designed to push your limits, helping you build strength, power, and endurance while testing your mental and physical resilience. As with all advanced training, it's important to listen to your body, maintain proper form, and rest adequately to avoid injury.

By incorporating these advanced techniques and HIIT into your workouts, you'll continue to challenge yourself and make significant strides in your fitness journey. Remember, consistency and dedication are key, so keep pushing your boundaries and enjoy the progress you make along the way.

Chapter 6: Targeted Workouts: Upper Body

A strong upper body not only enhances your physique but also improves your overall functional fitness, making everyday tasks easier and reducing the risk of injury. This chapter focuses on exercises that target the arms, shoulders, and back, using bodyweight, resistance bands, and dumbbells. We'll also provide an upper body circuit routine to help you sculpt and strengthen these key muscle groups.

Sculpting Your Arms, Shoulders, and Back

The upper body is made up of several major muscle groups, including the biceps, triceps, shoulders (deltoids), and the muscles of the upper back (trapezius, latissimus dorsi, and rhomboids). By targeting these areas, you can develop a balanced and well-defined upper body. Here are some effective exercises to get you started:

1. **Push-Ups:**
   -
   Muscles Targeted: Chest, shoulders, triceps
   -
   Instructions: Begin in a plank position with your hands slightly wider than shoulder-width apart. Lower your body until your chest nearly touches the floor, keeping your elbows close to your sides. Push back up to the starting position. For added difficulty, try decline push-ups or one-arm push-ups.
1. **Pull-Ups (or Inverted Rows):**
   -
   Muscles Targeted: Upper back, biceps, shoulders
   -
   Instructions: Grab a pull-up bar with an overhand grip, hands slightly wider than shoulder-width apart. Pull your body up until your chin clears the bar, then lower back down. If you don't have a pull-

up bar, inverted rows using a sturdy table or barbell on a rack are a great alternative.

1. **Dips:**
   -
     Muscles Targeted: Triceps, chest, shoulders
   -
     Instructions: Position yourself on parallel bars or between two sturdy surfaces, with your body upright and legs straight or bent. Lower your body by bending your elbows until your upper arms are parallel to the ground, then push back up to the starting position. This exercise can also be done using a chair or bench.
1. **Pike Push-Ups:**
   -
     Muscles Targeted: Shoulders, triceps
   -
     Instructions: Begin in a downward-facing dog position with your hips raised and body forming an inverted V. Lower your head towards the floor by bending your elbows, then push back up to the starting position. This exercise emphasizes the shoulders and mimics the motion of a handstand push-up.
1. **Plank Rows:**
   -
     Muscles Targeted: Back, shoulders, core
   -
     Instructions: Start in a plank position with a dumbbell in each hand. Keeping your core engaged, row one dumbbell up towards your waist, then lower it back to the floor. Repeat on the other side. This exercise can be done with just bodyweight by focusing on a controlled row motion.
1. **Superman:**
   -
     Muscles Targeted: Lower back, shoulders, glutes

o

Instructions: Lie face down on the floor with your arms extended in front of you. Lift your arms, chest, and legs off the ground simultaneously, squeezing your glutes and lower back muscles. Hold for a moment, then lower back down.

These exercises target all the major muscle groups in your upper body, helping you develop strength, endurance, and muscle definition. As you progress, you can increase the intensity by adding more repetitions, sets, or by incorporating resistance bands and dumbbells.

Resistance Bands and Dumbbells (If You Have Them)

If you have access to resistance bands or dumbbells, you can add variety and intensity to your upper body workouts. These tools allow you to perform a wider range of exercises and increase the resistance as you get stronger. Here are some effective exercises using resistance bands and dumbbells:

1. **Resistance Band Bicep Curls:**
   o
   Muscles Targeted: Biceps
   o
   Instructions: Stand on the middle of the resistance band with feet shoulder-width apart. Hold the ends of the band with your palms facing forward. Curl the band towards your shoulders, squeezing your biceps at the top, then slowly lower back down.
1. **Dumbbell Shoulder Press:**
   o
   Muscles Targeted: Shoulders (deltoids), triceps
   o
   Instructions: Hold a dumbbell in each hand at shoulder height, with your palms facing forward. Press the dumbbells overhead until your arms are

fully extended, then lower back down to shoulder height.

1. **Resistance Band Lat Pulldowns:**
   - **Muscles Targeted:** Upper back (latissimus dorsi)
   - **Instructions:** Secure a resistance band to a high anchor point. Sit or kneel, holding the band with both hands, arms extended overhead. Pull the band down towards your chest, squeezing your shoulder blades together, then slowly return to the starting position.

1. **Dumbbell Tricep Kickbacks:**
   - **Muscles Targeted:** Triceps
   - **Instructions:** Hold a dumbbell in each hand, hinge forward at the hips with a slight bend in the knees. Keep your upper arms close to your body and extend the dumbbells back, straightening your arms. Squeeze your triceps at the top, then slowly lower back down.

1. **Resistance Band Face Pulls:**
   - **Muscles Targeted:** Upper back, shoulders
   - **Instructions:** Attach a resistance band to a sturdy anchor at face height. Hold the band with both hands, arms extended in front of you. Pull the band towards your face, keeping your elbows high and squeezing your shoulder blades together, then slowly return to the starting position.

1. **Dumbbell Bent-Over Rows:**
   - **Muscles Targeted:** Upper back, shoulders, biceps
   -

Instructions: Hold a dumbbell in each hand, hinge forward at the hips with a slight bend in the knees. Keep your back flat and row the dumbbells towards your waist, squeezing your shoulder blades together. Lower the weights back down with control.

These exercises add resistance to your routine, helping you build muscle and strength more effectively. Resistance bands are particularly useful for those who want to train on the go or have limited space, while dumbbells allow for more traditional strength training.

Upper Body Circuit Routine

This upper body circuit routine combines bodyweight exercises with resistance band and dumbbell exercises to provide a comprehensive workout that targets all major muscle groups in the upper body. Perform this routine 2-3 times per week for best results.

Warm-Up (5 Minutes):

- **Arm Circles:** 1 minute (30 seconds each direction)
- **Jumping Jacks:** 1 minute
- **Push-Up Shoulder Taps:** 1 minute
- **Torso Twists:** 1 minute
- **Resistance Band Pull-Aparts:** 1 minute

Circuit: Complete each exercise for the prescribed number of repetitions, moving from one exercise to the next with minimal rest. After completing one full circuit, rest for 1-2 minutes, then repeat for a total of 3-4 rounds.

1. **Push-Ups:**
   - **Reps:** 12-15
   - **Instructions:** Perform standard or decline push-ups as described earlier.
1. **Resistance Band Lat Pulldowns:**
   - **Reps:** 12-15
   - **Instructions:** Perform lat pulldowns as described earlier.
1. **Dumbbell Shoulder Press:**
   - **Reps:** 10-12
   - **Instructions:** Perform shoulder presses as described earlier.
1. **Pull-Ups or Inverted Rows:**
   - **Reps:** 8-10
   - **Instructions:** Perform pull-ups or inverted rows as described earlier.
1. **Dips:**
   - **Reps:** 12-15
   - **Instructions:** Perform dips using parallel bars, a bench, or a chair.
1. **Resistance Band Bicep Curls:**
   - **Reps:** 12-15
   -

Instructions: Perform bicep curls as described earlier.

1. **Dumbbell Tricep Kickbacks:**
   - **Reps:** 12-15
   - **Instructions:** Perform tricep kickbacks as described earlier.
1. **Pike Push-Ups:**
   - **Reps:** 8-10
   -

   Instructions: Perform pike push-ups as described earlier.

Cool-Down (5 Minutes):

- **Shoulder Stretch:** 30 seconds per side
- **Tricep Stretch:** 30 seconds per side
- **Chest Stretch:** 1 minute
- **Child's Pose:** 1 minute
-

   Upper Back Stretch (Cat-Cow Pose): 1 minute

This circuit routine is designed to challenge your upper body muscles, building strength, endurance, and definition. By consistently incorporating these exercises into your fitness regimen, you'll develop a strong, balanced, and sculpted upper body.

Targeting the upper body with specific exercises not only enhances your appearance but also contributes to better overall functional strength and stability. Whether you're using just your bodyweight or incorporating resistance bands and dumbbells, these routines will help you achieve a stronger, more defined upper body.

Chapter 7: Targeted Workouts: Lower Body

A strong lower body is the foundation for overall fitness, supporting daily activities, enhancing athletic performance, and helping to prevent injuries. This chapter focuses on exercises that target the legs and glutes, providing options for bodyweight training as well as routines that incorporate minimal equipment. Additionally, you'll find a comprehensive lower body circuit routine to help you build strength, endurance, and muscle definition in your lower half.

Strengthening Your Legs and Glutes

The lower body consists of several major muscle groups, including the quadriceps, hamstrings, glutes, calves, and hip flexors. Strengthening these muscles not only improves your overall fitness but also contributes to better posture, balance, and mobility. Here are some key exercises to target each of these areas:

1. **Squats:**
   - **Muscles Targeted:** Quadriceps, glutes, hamstrings
   - **Instructions:** Stand with your feet shoulder-width apart, toes slightly turned out. Lower your body as if sitting back into a chair, keeping your chest up and knees tracking over your toes. Push through your heels to return to the starting position. Variations include sumo squats (wider stance) and pulse squats (holding a low position and pulsing).
1. **Lunges:**
   - **Muscles Targeted:** Quadriceps, glutes, hamstrings
   - **Instructions:** Stand with your feet together. Step forward with one leg and lower your body until both knees are bent at 90 degrees. Push through the

front heel to return to the starting position, then switch legs. Variations include reverse lunges, walking lunges, and lateral lunges.

1. **Glute Bridges:**
   - **Muscles Targeted:** Glutes, hamstrings, lower back
   - **Instructions:** Lie on your back with your knees bent and feet flat on the floor, hip-width apart. Lift your hips towards the ceiling, squeezing your glutes at the top. Lower your hips back down without touching the floor, and repeat. For added difficulty, try single-leg glute bridges.
1. **Step-Ups:**
   - **Muscles Targeted:** Quadriceps, glutes, calves
   - **Instructions:** Stand in front of a sturdy bench or step. Step up with one foot, pressing through the heel to lift your body onto the step. Step down and repeat on the other leg. This exercise can be intensified by holding dumbbells or adding a knee raise at the top.
1. **Calf Raises:**
   - **Muscles Targeted:** Calves
   - **Instructions:** Stand with your feet hip-width apart, either flat on the floor or on an elevated surface (like a step). Rise onto the balls of your feet, squeezing your calves at the top, then slowly lower back down. For added challenge, perform single-leg calf raises.
1. **Deadlifts (Bodyweight or Dumbbell):**
   - **Muscles Targeted:** Hamstrings, glutes, lower back
   -

Instructions: Stand with your feet hip-width apart, knees slightly bent. Hinge at the hips to lower your torso towards the ground while keeping your back straight. If using dumbbells, hold them in front of your thighs and lower them towards the floor. Squeeze your glutes as you return to the starting position.

These exercises target the major muscles of the lower body, helping you build strength, improve endurance, and develop greater muscle definition. Whether you're using just your bodyweight or incorporating equipment, these movements are essential for a well-rounded fitness routine.

Bodyweight and Minimal Equipment Options

Training your lower body effectively doesn't require a gym full of equipment. Bodyweight exercises can be highly effective, and adding minimal equipment like resistance bands or dumbbells can further enhance your workouts. Here are some bodyweight and minimal equipment options for lower body training:

1. **Bodyweight Squats and Variations:**
   - **Instructions:** Squats can be performed using just your bodyweight, with variations such as sumo squats, pulse squats, or jump squats to increase intensity.
1. **Resistance Band Glute Bridges:**
   - **Instructions:** Place a resistance band around your thighs just above your knees. Perform glute bridges as described earlier, pressing against the band to add resistance and engage your glutes more effectively.
1. **Single-Leg Deadlifts:**
   -

Instructions: Hold a dumbbell in one hand (or use just bodyweight) and perform a deadlift while lifting the opposite leg behind you. This variation targets the hamstrings and glutes while improving balance and stability.

1. **Wall Sits:**
   - **Instructions:** Stand with your back against a wall and slide down until your knees are bent at 90 degrees, as if sitting in an invisible chair. Hold this position for as long as possible, engaging your quads, glutes, and core.
1. **Bulgarian Split Squats:**
   - **Instructions:** Stand a few feet in front of a bench or chair, with one foot resting on the surface behind you. Perform a lunge, lowering your back knee towards the floor, then push through the front heel to return to the starting position. This exercise can be intensified by holding dumbbells.
1. **Resistance Band Kickbacks:**
   - **Instructions:** Attach a resistance band to a sturdy anchor and around one ankle. Stand facing the anchor and kick the banded leg straight back, squeezing your glutes at the top. Return to the starting position and repeat on the other leg.

By incorporating these bodyweight and minimal equipment options into your routine, you can effectively target your lower body muscles, build strength, and improve muscle tone—all from the comfort of your home.

Lower Body Circuit Routine

This lower body circuit routine combines bodyweight exercises with optional resistance band and dumbbell exercises to create a comprehensive workout that targets all major muscle groups in the lower body. Perform this routine 2-3 times per week, with at least one rest day between sessions.

Warm-Up (5 Minutes):

- **Jumping Jacks or High Knees:** 1 minute
- **Leg Swings:** 30 seconds per leg
- **Bodyweight Squats:** 1 minute
- **Hip Circles:** 30 seconds each direction
- **Calf Raises:** 1 minute

Circuit: Complete each exercise for the prescribed number of repetitions, moving from one exercise to the next with minimal rest. After completing one full circuit, rest for 1-2 minutes, then repeat for a total of 3-4 rounds.

1. **Squats or Sumo Squats:**
   - **Reps:** 15-20
   - **Instructions:** Perform bodyweight squats or sumo squats as described earlier. For added intensity, hold a dumbbell or perform jump squats.
1. **Lunges or Bulgarian Split Squats:**
   - **Reps:** 12-15 per leg
   - **Instructions:** Perform lunges or Bulgarian split squats as described earlier. Hold dumbbells or add a knee raise for added difficulty.

1. **Glute Bridges or Resistance Band Glute Bridges:**
   - **Reps:** 15-20
   - **Instructions:** Perform glute bridges or resistance band glute bridges as described earlier. Squeeze your glutes at the top of each rep.
1. **Step-Ups:**
   - **Reps:** 12-15 per leg
   - **Instructions:** Perform step-ups as described earlier. Hold dumbbells or add a knee raise for added challenge.
1. **Deadlifts (Bodyweight, Dumbbell, or Single-Leg):**
   - **Reps:** 12-15
   - **Instructions:** Perform deadlifts as described earlier, choosing the variation that best suits your fitness level.
1. **Wall Sits:**
   - **Time:** 30-60 seconds
   - **Instructions:** Perform wall sits as described earlier, holding the position for as long as possible.
1. **Calf Raises or Single-Leg Calf Raises:**
   - **Reps:** 15-20
   - **Instructions:** Perform calf raises or single-leg calf raises as described earlier. Hold the top position for a brief pause to increase the intensity.

Cool-Down (5 Minutes):

- **Hamstring Stretch:** 30 seconds per leg
- **Quad Stretch:** 30 seconds per leg
- **Glute Stretch (Figure Four Stretch):** 30 seconds per side
- **Hip Flexor Stretch:** 30 seconds per side
- **Calf Stretch:** 30 seconds per leg

This circuit routine is designed to challenge your lower body muscles, build strength and endurance, and improve muscle tone. By consistently incorporating these exercises into your fitness regimen, you'll develop stronger, more defined legs and glutes.

Strengthening your lower body is crucial for overall fitness and functional movement. Whether you're using just your bodyweight or incorporating minimal equipment, these targeted exercises and routines will help you achieve a strong, balanced, and powerful lower body.

Chapter 8: Core Strengthening Workouts

A strong core is the foundation of a fit and healthy body. It plays a crucial role in almost every movement you make, from simple daily activities to complex athletic maneuvers. This chapter will delve into the importance of a strong core, introduce you to exercises that enhance core stability and strength, and provide a core-focused workout routine to help you develop a solid and functional core.

The Importance of a Strong Core

Your core muscles, which include the abdominals, obliques, lower back, and hip muscles, are responsible for stabilizing your spine, supporting your posture, and transferring force between your upper and lower body. A strong core offers numerous benefits, including:

1. **Improved Posture:**
   - A strong core helps you maintain proper posture, reducing the strain on your spine and preventing issues like back pain. Good posture also enhances your appearance and can even boost your confidence.
1. **Enhanced Balance and Stability:**
   - Core strength is essential for maintaining balance and stability, whether you're standing still, moving through space, or performing complex exercises. A stable core allows you to control your movements more effectively and reduces the risk of falls and injuries.
1. **Increased Functional Strength:**
   - Many everyday activities, such as lifting, bending, and twisting, rely on a strong core. A well-

developed core improves your ability to perform these tasks with greater ease and efficiency.

1. **Better Athletic Performance:**
   -

   Athletes across all sports benefit from a strong core, as it enhances their ability to generate power, maintain balance, and prevent injuries. Whether you're running, jumping, or throwing, a strong core is key to maximizing your performance.

1. **Injury Prevention:**
   -

   A strong core helps to stabilize your spine and pelvis, reducing the risk of lower back pain and other injuries. It also protects your body during sudden movements or impacts by providing a solid foundation of support.

1. **Improved Breathing and Circulation:**
   -

   The muscles of the core are involved in breathing and circulation. A strong core can improve your breathing efficiency and promote better blood flow throughout your body.

Given its critical role in overall fitness and health, it's essential to regularly incorporate core-strengthening exercises into your workout routine.

Core Exercises for Stability and Strength

Core exercises can be divided into two categories: stability exercises, which focus on maintaining balance and control, and strength exercises, which focus on building muscle and power. Here are some of the most effective exercises for each category:

1. **Plank:**
   -
   - **Type:** Stability

○

Instructions: Begin in a forearm plank position with your body in a straight line from head to heels. Engage your core, avoiding sagging or arching your back. Hold this position for as long as possible, focusing on maintaining proper form.

1. **Side Plank:**

   ○

   Type: Stability

   ○

   Instructions: Lie on your side with your legs straight and your forearm directly under your shoulder. Lift your hips off the ground, creating a straight line from head to feet. Hold this position, engaging your obliques and core. Repeat on the other side.

1. **Dead Bug:**

   ○

   Type: Stability

   ○

   Instructions: Lie on your back with your arms extended towards the ceiling and your knees bent at 90 degrees. Slowly lower your right arm and left leg towards the floor while keeping your lower back pressed into the ground. Return to the starting position and repeat on the other side. This exercise enhances core stability and coordination.

1. **Russian Twists:**

   ○

   Type: Strength

   ○

   Instructions: Sit on the floor with your knees bent and feet lifted off the ground. Hold your hands together in front of you or a weight (like a dumbbell or medicine ball). Twist your torso to one side, bringing your hands or the weight towards the floor, then twist to the other side. This exercise targets the obliques and improves rotational strength.

1. **Leg Raises:**
   - **Type:** Strength
   - **Instructions:** Lie on your back with your legs straight and arms by your sides. Lift your legs towards the ceiling, keeping them straight, until they form a 90-degree angle with your torso. Slowly lower them back down without letting them touch the floor. This exercise targets the lower abdominals.
1. **Bicycle Crunches:**
   - **Type:** Strength
   - **Instructions:** Lie on your back with your hands behind your head and legs lifted off the ground. Bring your right elbow towards your left knee while extending your right leg. Switch sides, bringing your left elbow towards your right knee. Continue alternating in a pedaling motion. This exercise targets the obliques and the entire abdominal region.
1. **Mountain Climbers:**
   - **Type:** Strength and Stability
   - **Instructions:** Begin in a plank position. Quickly alternate bringing one knee towards your chest, then switch to the other, as if running in place. This exercise targets the core, shoulders, and legs, providing both a strength and cardio challenge.
1. **Superman:**
   - **Type:** Strength

○

Instructions: Lie face down on the floor with your arms extended in front of you. Lift your arms, chest, and legs off the ground simultaneously, squeezing your lower back and glutes. Hold for a moment, then lower back down. This exercise targets the lower back, glutes, and core.

These exercises cover all aspects of core training, from building stability and balance to developing strength and endurance. Incorporate a mix of these movements into your routine to create a well-rounded core workout.

Core-Focused Workout Routine

This core-focused workout routine is designed to target all major muscle groups in your core, helping you build strength, stability, and endurance. Perform this routine 2-3 times per week, either as a standalone workout or as part of a full-body training session.

Warm-Up (5 Minutes):

- **Cat-Cow Stretch:** 1 minute
- **Torso Twists:** 1 minute
- **Leg Swings:** 30 seconds per leg
- **Hip Circles:** 1 minute
- **Jumping Jacks:** 1 minute

Workout: Complete each exercise for the prescribed number of repetitions or duration, moving from one exercise to the next with minimal rest. After completing one full circuit, rest for 1-2 minutes, then repeat for a total of 3-4 rounds.

1. **Plank:**
   - **Time:** 30-60 seconds
   - **Instructions:** Hold the plank position as described earlier. Focus on keeping your core tight and your body in a straight line.
1. **Russian Twists:**
   - **Reps:** 20-30 twists (10-15 per side)
   - **Instructions:** Perform Russian twists as described earlier, using a weight if desired for added resistance.
1. **Dead Bug:**
   - **Reps:** 10-12 per side
   - **Instructions:** Perform the dead bug exercise as described earlier, focusing on maintaining stability and control.
1. **Leg Raises:**
   - **Reps:** 12-15
   - **Instructions:** Perform leg raises as described earlier, keeping your core engaged and your movements slow and controlled.
1. **Side Plank:**
   - **Time:** 20-30 seconds per side
   -

Instructions: Hold the side plank position as described earlier, ensuring your body forms a straight line from head to feet.

1. **Bicycle Crunches:**
   - **Reps:** 20-30 (10-15 per side)
   - **Instructions:** Perform bicycle crunches as described earlier, focusing on engaging your core and twisting from your torso.
1. **Mountain Climbers:**
   - **Time:** 30-45 seconds
   - **Instructions:** Perform mountain climbers as described earlier, maintaining a steady pace and keeping your core tight.
1. **Superman:**
   - **Reps:** 12-15
   -

   Instructions: Perform the Superman exercise as described earlier, holding the top position for a brief pause before lowering back down.

Cool-Down (5 Minutes):

- **Child's Pose:** 1 minute
- **Cobra Stretch:** 1 minute
- **Seated Forward Bend:** 1 minute
- **Spinal Twist:** 30 seconds per side
-

Hip Flexor Stretch: 1 minute (30 seconds per side)

This core-focused workout routine is designed to challenge and strengthen your entire core, helping you build a solid foundation for overall fitness. By regularly incorporating these exercises into your training regimen, you'll develop a strong, stable, and functional core that supports every aspect of your physical activity.

Developing a strong core is essential for overall fitness, injury prevention, and improved athletic performance. With this comprehensive approach to core strengthening, you'll be well on your way to achieving a powerful, resilient core that enhances your quality of life and supports your fitness goals.

Chapter 9: Cardio Workouts You Can Do Anywhere

Cardiovascular exercise, or cardio, is essential for maintaining heart health, improving endurance, and burning calories. The beauty of cardio is that it can be done virtually anywhere, often with no equipment needed. This chapter explores various no-equipment cardio options, discusses how to combine cardio with strength training for a well-rounded workout, and provides a cardio circuit routine you can perform at home, in a park, or wherever you find yourself.

No-Equipment Cardio Options

Cardio workouts don't require fancy machines or equipment. Many effective exercises use only your bodyweight, making them accessible and convenient no matter where you are. Here are some no-equipment cardio exercises that are simple yet powerful:

1. **Jumping Jacks:**
   - **Instructions:** Stand with your feet together and arms at your sides. Jump your feet out to the sides while raising your arms overhead, then quickly return to the starting position. This classic move gets your heart rate up quickly and engages multiple muscle groups.
1. **High Knees:**
   - **Instructions:** Stand in place and run by bringing your knees up towards your chest as high as possible. Pump your arms as you move, maintaining a quick pace. High knees are excellent for boosting cardiovascular endurance and working your core.
1. **Burpees:**
   -

Instructions: From a standing position, drop into a squat and place your hands on the floor. Jump your feet back into a plank position, perform a push-up, then jump your feet back to your hands and explode into a jump. Burpees provide a full-body workout and elevate your heart rate quickly.

1. **Mountain Climbers:**
   - **Instructions:** Start in a plank position. Quickly alternate bringing one knee towards your chest, then switch to the other, as if running in place. Mountain climbers target your core, shoulders, and legs while providing a great cardio challenge.

1. **Jump Squats:**
   - **Instructions:** Perform a regular squat, but as you stand up, explode into a jump, reaching your arms overhead. Land softly and immediately lower into the next squat. Jump squats build lower body strength while increasing your heart rate.

1. **Butt Kicks:**
   - **Instructions:** Stand in place and run by kicking your heels up towards your glutes with each step. Keep a fast pace and use your arms to maintain rhythm. Butt kicks are great for warming up or as part of a high-intensity interval.

1. **Shadow Boxing:**
   - **Instructions:** Stand in a fighting stance with your feet shoulder-width apart and hands up in front of your face. Throw punches (jabs, crosses, hooks) into the air while moving your feet. Shadow boxing is a fun way to incorporate cardio while improving coordination and agility.

1. **Skaters:**
   -

Instructions: Stand with your feet hip-width apart. Jump to the right, landing on your right foot while sweeping your left leg behind your right. Jump to the left, landing on your left foot while sweeping your right leg behind. Skaters mimic the motion of speed skating and improve lateral movement, balance, and coordination.

These exercises can be mixed and matched to create a variety of cardio routines, making it easy to stay engaged and avoid monotony. They require no equipment and can be done in small spaces, making them ideal for home workouts or on-the-go fitness.

Combining Cardio with Strength Training

Combining cardio with strength training in the same workout is an efficient way to burn calories, build muscle, and improve overall fitness. This approach not only maximizes your workout time but also creates a balanced routine that targets multiple aspects of physical fitness. Here's how you can effectively combine cardio and strength training:

1. **Circuit Training:**
   - **Description:** Circuit training involves performing a series of exercises back-to-back with minimal rest in between. By alternating between cardio and strength exercises, you can keep your heart rate elevated while building muscle. For example, you might alternate between push-ups, jumping jacks, squats, and burpees in a single circuit.
1. **HIIT (High-Intensity Interval Training):**
   - **Description:** HIIT involves short bursts of intense exercise followed by brief periods of rest. By incorporating both cardio and strength moves into a HIIT session, you can improve cardiovascular fitness while building strength. An example might

be 30 seconds of mountain climbers followed by 30 seconds of push-ups, repeated for several rounds.

1. **Cardio with Bodyweight Exercises:**
   -

   Description: Bodyweight exercises such as squats, lunges, and push-ups can be incorporated into a cardio routine to enhance strength while keeping the heart rate up. For instance, you might perform 10 squats followed by 30 seconds of high knees, then move on to another strength exercise paired with a cardio move.

1. **Supersets:**
   -

   Description: Supersets involve performing two exercises back-to-back with no rest in between. By pairing a strength exercise with a cardio move, you can keep your heart rate elevated throughout the workout. For example, a superset might include 12 reps of dumbbell rows followed immediately by 30 seconds of jump rope.

1. **Plyometrics:**
   -

   Description: Plyometric exercises, which involve explosive movements like jumping, are a great way to combine strength and cardio. Moves like jump squats, burpees, and box jumps build power and strength while providing a cardiovascular challenge.

By combining cardio and strength training, you create a comprehensive workout that improves both aerobic and anaerobic fitness, enhances muscle tone, and promotes fat loss. This approach is ideal for those who want to maximize their workout efficiency and achieve balanced fitness results.

Cardio Circuit Routine

This cardio circuit routine is designed to elevate your heart rate, improve cardiovascular fitness, and burn calories, all while engaging your muscles with strength and endurance exercises. Perform this routine 2-3 times per week for optimal results.

Warm-Up (5 Minutes):

- **Jump Rope or High Knees:** 1 minute
- **Arm Circles:** 30 seconds each direction
- **Leg Swings:** 30 seconds per leg
- **Torso Twists:** 1 minute
- **Lateral Shuffles:** 1 minute

Circuit: Complete each exercise for the prescribed time or repetitions, moving from one exercise to the next with minimal rest. After completing one full circuit, rest for 1-2 minutes, then repeat for a total of 3-4 rounds.

1. **Jumping Jacks:**
   - **Time:** 45 seconds
   - **Instructions:** Perform jumping jacks as described earlier, maintaining a steady pace.
1. **Push-Ups:**
   - **Reps:** 12-15
   - **Instructions:** Perform standard push-ups, decline push-ups, or knee push-ups depending on your fitness level.
1. **High Knees:**

o

Time: 45 seconds

o

Instructions: Perform high knees as described earlier, driving your knees up towards your chest with each step.

1. **Bodyweight Squats:**

   o

   Reps: 15-20

   o

   Instructions: Perform bodyweight squats, focusing on depth and control. Add a jump at the top for increased intensity.

1. **Mountain Climbers:**

   o

   Time: 45 seconds

   o

   Instructions: Perform mountain climbers as described earlier, keeping your core engaged and maintaining a quick pace.

1. **Plank to Push-Up:**

   o

   Reps: 10-12

   o

   Instructions: Start in a forearm plank position. Push up onto your hands, one hand at a time, until you're in a full plank position. Lower back down to the forearm plank and repeat.

1. **Burpees:**

   o

   Reps: 10-12

   o

   Instructions: Perform burpees as described earlier, focusing on maintaining a steady rhythm throughout the movement.

1. **Lunges (Walking or Stationary):**

   o

Reps: 12-15 per leg

o

Instructions: Perform walking lunges or stationary lunges, ensuring your front knee is aligned with your ankle.

1. **Skaters:**

   o

   Time: 45 seconds

   o

   Instructions: Perform skaters as described earlier, jumping from side to side with control and balance.

Cool-Down (5 Minutes):

- **Hamstring Stretch:** 30 seconds per leg
- **Quad Stretch:** 30 seconds per leg
- **Calf Stretch:** 30 seconds per leg
- **Chest Stretch:** 30 seconds
- **Child's Pose:** 1 minute

This cardio circuit routine provides a balanced workout that combines high-intensity cardiovascular exercises with bodyweight strength movements. It's designed to improve overall fitness, burn calories, and enhance endurance, making it a valuable addition to your workout regimen.

Incorporating cardio workouts into your routine is essential for maintaining a healthy heart, improving endurance, and burning calories. Whether you're doing no-equipment exercises, combining cardio with strength training, or following a structured circuit, these workouts can be done anywhere, making it easier than ever to stay fit and active.

Chapter 10: Flexibility and Mobility Exercises

Flexibility and mobility are often overlooked components of fitness, but they play a crucial role in maintaining overall health, preventing injuries, and enhancing physical performance. This chapter explores the importance of flexibility in fitness, introduces yoga and stretching routines designed to improve flexibility, and provides a daily mobility routine to keep your body moving freely and efficiently.

The Role of Flexibility in Fitness

Flexibility refers to the ability of your muscles and joints to move through their full range of motion. It is a key component of overall fitness and contributes to several aspects of physical health and performance:

1. **Improved Range of Motion:**
   - Flexibility allows your joints to move more freely, which can improve your performance in various activities, from daily tasks to athletic pursuits. A greater range of motion can enhance your ability to perform exercises with proper form, reducing the risk of injury.
1. **Injury Prevention:**
   - Flexible muscles are less prone to strains and tears. By improving flexibility, you reduce the likelihood of sustaining injuries during physical activities. Stretching helps to keep muscles pliable and reduces tension, which can decrease the risk of muscle pulls and other injuries.
1. **Enhanced Posture:**
   - Flexibility, particularly in the muscles of the back, shoulders, and hips, plays a significant role in

maintaining good posture. Tight muscles can lead to poor alignment, which can cause discomfort and long-term issues. Regular stretching helps to maintain proper posture and alignment, reducing the strain on your body.

1. **Better Circulation:**
   - Stretching improves blood flow to the muscles, which can enhance recovery after exercise and promote overall muscle health. Increased circulation also helps to remove waste products from the muscles, reducing soreness and stiffness.

1. **Reduced Muscle Tension and Stress:**
   - Flexibility exercises can help relieve muscle tension and reduce stress. Stretching, particularly when combined with deep breathing, can calm the nervous system, leading to a greater sense of relaxation and well-being.

1. **Improved Athletic Performance:**
   -

   Athletes often incorporate flexibility training to improve their performance. Enhanced flexibility can lead to better movement efficiency, greater power output, and reduced fatigue during activities.

Given the numerous benefits of flexibility, it's essential to incorporate regular stretching and mobility exercises into your fitness routine. This will not only improve your physical performance but also contribute to your overall health and well-being.

Yoga and Stretching Routines for Flexibility

Yoga and stretching routines are excellent ways to improve flexibility, as they involve gentle, controlled movements that lengthen the muscles and increase joint mobility. Here are some key yoga poses and stretching exercises to incorporate into your routine:

1. **Downward-Facing Dog (Adho Mukha Svanasana):**
   - **Instructions:** Start on your hands and knees, then lift your hips towards the ceiling, forming an inverted V shape with your body. Keep your hands shoulder-width apart and your feet hip-width apart. Press your heels towards the ground and lengthen your spine. This pose stretches the hamstrings, calves, and shoulders, while also improving overall flexibility.
1. **Cobra Pose (Bhujangasana):**
   - **Instructions:** Lie face down on the floor with your hands under your shoulders. Press into your hands to lift your chest off the ground, keeping your elbows slightly bent and your shoulders away from your ears. This pose stretches the chest, shoulders, and abdominal muscles, while also improving spinal flexibility.
1. **Seated Forward Bend (Paschimottanasana):**
   - **Instructions:** Sit with your legs extended straight in front of you. Inhale and lengthen your spine, then exhale as you hinge at the hips to reach towards your toes. Keep your back straight and focus on stretching the hamstrings and lower back. This pose enhances flexibility in the posterior chain, including the hamstrings and spine.
1. **Butterfly Stretch:**
   - **Instructions:** Sit with your feet together and your knees bent, allowing your knees to fall open to the sides. Hold your feet with your hands and gently

press your knees towards the ground. This stretch targets the inner thighs and hips, improving flexibility in the groin area.

1. **Standing Forward Bend (Uttanasana):**
   -

   Instructions: Stand with your feet hip-width apart. Inhale and lift your arms overhead, then exhale as you hinge at the hips to fold forward, reaching towards the ground or your ankles. Allow your head to hang heavy and relax your neck. This pose stretches the hamstrings, calves, and lower back, while also promoting relaxation.

1. **Child's Pose (Balasana):**
   -

   Instructions: Kneel on the floor with your big toes touching and your knees spread wide. Sit back on your heels and extend your arms forward, lowering your chest towards the ground. Rest your forehead on the floor and breathe deeply. This pose gently stretches the lower back, hips, and thighs, while promoting relaxation and stress relief.

1. **Cat-Cow Stretch:**
   -

   Instructions: Start on your hands and knees in a tabletop position. Inhale as you arch your back, lifting your head and tailbone towards the ceiling (Cow Pose). Exhale as you round your spine, tucking your chin towards your chest and bringing your tailbone towards your knees (Cat Pose). This dynamic stretch improves flexibility in the spine and helps to alleviate tension.

These yoga poses and stretches can be performed as part of a dedicated flexibility routine or incorporated into your cool-down after a workout. Aim to hold each pose for 30 seconds to a minute, breathing deeply and allowing your muscles to relax into the stretch.

Daily Mobility Routine

In addition to flexibility, mobility is essential for maintaining healthy joints and muscles. Mobility exercises focus on improving the movement and function of your joints, ensuring they move smoothly through their full range of motion. A daily mobility routine can help you stay active, prevent stiffness, and enhance your overall physical performance. Here's a simple daily mobility routine to keep your body moving freely:

1. **Hip Circles:**
   - **Instructions:** Stand with your feet hip-width apart and place your hands on your hips. Slowly rotate your hips in a circular motion, making large circles in one direction for 30 seconds, then switch to the other direction. This exercise improves hip mobility and loosens the lower back.
1. **Shoulder Rolls:**
   - **Instructions:** Stand with your feet shoulder-width apart and your arms relaxed at your sides. Slowly roll your shoulders forward in a circular motion for 30 seconds, then reverse the direction and roll them backward. This exercise improves shoulder mobility and relieves tension in the upper back and neck.
1. **Thoracic Spine Rotations:**
   - **Instructions:** Sit or stand with your hands clasped behind your head. Rotate your torso to the right, keeping your hips stable, then return to the center and rotate to the left. Perform 10-12 rotations on

each side. This exercise improves mobility in the thoracic spine and enhances rotational movement.

1. **Ankle Circles:**
   - **Instructions:** Sit or stand with one leg lifted off the ground. Slowly rotate your ankle in a circular motion, making large circles in one direction for 15 seconds, then switch to the other direction. Repeat with the other ankle. This exercise improves ankle mobility and helps prevent stiffness.

1. **World's Greatest Stretch:**
   - **Instructions:** Start in a lunge position with your right foot forward and your left leg extended back. Place your left hand on the ground and twist your torso to the right, reaching your right hand towards the ceiling. Hold for a few seconds, then switch sides. This exercise improves mobility in the hips, spine, and shoulders.

1. **Scapular Push-Ups:**
   - **Instructions:** Start in a plank position with your arms straight and hands under your shoulders. Without bending your elbows, squeeze your shoulder blades together, then push them apart as you return to the starting position. Perform 10-12 reps. This exercise improves shoulder stability and mobility.

1. **Lunge with Overhead Reach:**
   - **Instructions:** Step forward into a lunge with your right foot, while raising your left arm overhead and reaching towards the ceiling. Hold for a few seconds, then return to the starting position and switch sides. This exercise improves mobility in the hips, shoulders, and spine.

1. **Neck Tilts:**

○

Instructions: Stand or sit with your back straight. Slowly tilt your head to the right, bringing your ear towards your shoulder, and hold for a few seconds. Return to the center and repeat on the left side. Perform 5-6 tilts on each side. This exercise improves neck mobility and relieves tension.

This daily mobility routine takes just a few minutes to complete and can be done in the morning to wake up your body, during the day to relieve stiffness, or as part of your cool-down after a workout. Regularly practicing these mobility exercises will help keep your joints healthy, improve your movement efficiency, and reduce the risk of injury.

Flexibility and mobility are essential components of a well-rounded fitness routine. By incorporating yoga, stretching, and mobility exercises into your daily regimen, you'll enhance your overall physical performance, reduce the risk of injury, and enjoy greater freedom of movement in your everyday life.

Chapter 11: Creating Custom Workout Plans

Crafting a workout plan tailored to your specific goals, preferences, and fitness level is one of the most effective ways to ensure consistent progress and long-term success. In this chapter, you'll learn how to mix and match exercises to create balanced routines, design a weekly workout schedule that fits your lifestyle, and adapt your plan as you progress. By the end, you'll have the tools to create a custom workout plan that keeps you motivated, challenged, and on track to achieving your fitness goals.

How to Mix and Match Exercises

One of the key aspects of creating a custom workout plan is knowing how to mix and match exercises to target different muscle groups, improve overall fitness, and prevent boredom. Here's how to structure your workouts effectively:

1. **Identify Your Goals:**
   - Before selecting exercises, clearly define your fitness goals. Are you looking to build muscle, lose fat, improve endurance, or enhance flexibility? Your goals will determine the types of exercises you prioritize in your routine.
1. **Choose a Workout Format:**
   - Decide on the structure of your workouts. Common formats include:
     - **Full-Body Workouts:** Target all major muscle groups in a single session. Ideal for beginners or those with limited time to work out.
     - **Split Routines:** Focus on specific muscle groups on different days (e.g., upper body

on one day, lower body on another). This allows for more targeted training and recovery time.

- **Circuit Training:** Combine strength and cardio exercises in a fast-paced, circuit-style format. This is great for improving overall fitness and burning calories.

1. **Balance Muscle Groups:**
   - Ensure your workout plan targets all major muscle groups to create a balanced physique and prevent muscle imbalances. Include exercises for the following:
     - **Upper Body:** Chest, back, shoulders, biceps, triceps
     - **Lower Body:** Quads, hamstrings, glutes, calves
     - **Core:** Abdominals, obliques, lower back
     - **Cardio and Mobility:** Include exercises that improve cardiovascular health and flexibility.

1. **Select Exercises for Each Muscle Group:**
   - Choose a variety of exercises that target each muscle group from different angles. For example:
     - **Chest:** Push-ups, bench presses, chest flyes
     - **Back:** Pull-ups, rows, deadlifts
     - **Legs:** Squats, lunges, deadlifts

Shoulders: Shoulder presses, lateral raises, front raises

■

Core: Planks, Russian twists, leg raises

1. **Incorporate Different Types of Training:**
    o

    Mix in different types of training to keep your routine dynamic and challenging:

    ■

    Strength Training: Focus on lifting heavier weights or performing bodyweight exercises with higher resistance.

    ■

    Cardio Training: Include exercises like running, cycling, or jump rope to improve cardiovascular health.

    ■

    Flexibility and Mobility: Incorporate yoga, stretching, or foam rolling to improve flexibility and reduce muscle tension.

1. **Plan for Progression:**
    o

    Ensure your plan allows for progression by gradually increasing the intensity, volume, or complexity of your exercises. This could mean adding more weight, increasing the number of sets or reps, or trying more challenging variations of the exercises.

Designing a Weekly Workout Schedule

Once you've selected your exercises and determined your workout structure, it's time to design a weekly workout schedule that fits your lifestyle and helps you achieve your goals. Here's how to create an effective schedule:

1. **Determine Your Workout Frequency:**

o

Decide how many days per week you can commit to working out. For most people, 3-5 days per week is ideal for balancing effectiveness with recovery. Beginners might start with 3 days, while more advanced individuals might aim for 5-6 days.

1. **Assign Focus Areas to Each Day:**

   o

   Based on your chosen workout format (full-body, split routine, etc.), assign focus areas to each day. For example:

   - **3-Day Full-Body Schedule:**
     - Day 1: Full-Body Strength
     - Day 2: Cardio and Core
     - Day 3: Full-Body Strength

   - **4-Day Split Routine:**
     - Day 1: Upper Body Strength
     - Day 2: Lower Body Strength
     - Day 3: Cardio and Core
     - Day 4: Upper Body Strength

1. **Plan for Rest and Recovery:**

   o

   Schedule rest days or lighter activity days to allow your muscles to recover and prevent burnout. For example, if you're working out 5 days a week, you might rest on Day 4 and Day 7, or include active recovery activities like yoga or walking.

1. **Incorporate Variety:**

- ○

  Vary your workouts throughout the week to keep them engaging and to target your muscles from different angles. This could involve mixing strength training with cardio, changing up your exercises, or adjusting your workout intensity.

1. **Schedule Time for Flexibility and Mobility:**
   - ○

     Dedicate at least one session per week to flexibility and mobility exercises, or incorporate these into your daily routine. This helps prevent injuries, improves performance, and enhances overall well-being.

1. **Example Weekly Workout Schedule:**
   - ○

     Monday: Upper Body Strength
   - ○

     Tuesday: Lower Body Strength
   - ○

     Wednesday: Cardio and Core
   - ○

     Thursday: Rest or Active Recovery (e.g., yoga or walking)
   - ○

     Friday: Full-Body Strength
   - ○

     Saturday: Cardio and Flexibility
   - ○

     Sunday: Rest

This example schedule balances strength training with cardio and flexibility, allowing for sufficient recovery while targeting all major muscle groups.

Adapting Routines as You Progress

As you continue on your fitness journey, it's important to adapt your workout routine to reflect your progress and keep challenging your body. Here's how to adjust your plan as you improve:

1. **Monitor Your Progress:**
   - Keep track of your workouts, including the exercises you perform, the weights you use, the number of sets and reps, and how you feel during and after each session. This will help you identify areas where you're improving and areas that might need more focus.

1. **Increase Intensity:**
   - As your strength and endurance improve, gradually increase the intensity of your workouts. This can be done by:
     - **Adding Weight:** Increase the amount of weight you lift or the resistance you use for bodyweight exercises.
     - **Increasing Reps or Sets:** Add more repetitions or sets to your exercises as you build strength and stamina.
     - **Reducing Rest Time:** Shorten the rest periods between sets or exercises to keep your heart rate up and increase the challenge.
     - **Incorporating Advanced Exercises:** Try more complex or advanced variations of exercises to continue challenging your muscles.

1. **Switch Up Your Exercises:**
   -

Periodically change the exercises in your routine to prevent plateaus and keep your workouts interesting. For example, if you've been doing squats for a few weeks, try switching to lunges or step-ups to target your legs in a different way.

1. **Adjust Your Goals:**
    -

    As you reach your initial fitness goals, set new ones to keep yourself motivated and on track. Whether it's lifting a heavier weight, running a faster mile, or mastering a new exercise, having clear goals will help you stay focused and driven.

1. **Listen to Your Body:**
    -

    Pay attention to how your body feels and adjust your workouts accordingly. If you're feeling fatigued or experiencing pain, consider taking a rest day or focusing on lighter activities like stretching or yoga. Conversely, if you're feeling strong and energized, you might challenge yourself with a more intense workout.

1. **Periodization:**
    -

    Consider implementing periodization into your training plan. Periodization involves dividing your training into cycles (e.g., weeks or months) with varying intensity and focus. For example, you might have a strength-focused phase followed by an endurance-focused phase, helping you peak at the right times and avoid overtraining.

By adapting your workout plan as you progress, you'll continue to challenge your body, prevent plateaus, and achieve new levels of fitness. Remember that fitness is a journey, and it's important to stay flexible and open to changes as you grow and improve.

Creating a custom workout plan that aligns with your goals, fits your schedule, and adapts to your progress is key to achieving long-term fitness success. By mixing and matching exercises, designing a weekly workout schedule, and adjusting your routine as you improve, you'll stay motivated, avoid plateaus, and continue making strides towards your fitness goals.

Chapter 12: Staying Motivated and Consistent

One of the biggest challenges in any fitness journey is maintaining motivation and consistency over the long term. Even with the best workout plan, it's easy to lose momentum, encounter plateaus, or simply feel bored. This chapter provides practical tips for building a sustainable workout habit, overcoming plateaus, and keeping your workouts fun and engaging to ensure you stay on track towards your fitness goals.

Tips for Building a Workout Habit

Building a consistent workout habit is crucial for long-term success. The following strategies will help you make exercise a regular part of your life:

1. **Set Clear, Achievable Goals:**
    - Start with specific, measurable, and realistic goals that are meaningful to you. Whether it's losing weight, building muscle, or running a 5K, having clear objectives will give you a sense of direction and purpose.
1. **Create a Routine:**
    - Establish a regular workout schedule that fits your lifestyle. Consistency is key, so choose days and times when you can realistically commit to exercise. Over time, working out at the same time each day will become a habit.
1. **Start Small and Build Gradually:**
    - If you're new to exercise or returning after a break, start with manageable workouts. Gradually increase the intensity, duration, and frequency of your sessions as you build strength and endurance. This approach helps prevent burnout and injury.

1. **Find an Accountability Partner:**
   - Working out with a friend, family member, or joining a fitness group can provide motivation and accountability. Having someone to share your journey with makes exercise more enjoyable and helps you stay committed.
1. **Track Your Progress:**
   - Keep a workout journal or use a fitness app to record your workouts, track your progress, and celebrate your achievements. Seeing tangible results, like increased strength or improved endurance, can boost motivation and encourage you to keep going.
1. **Reward Yourself:**
   - Set up a reward system for reaching milestones, such as treating yourself to new workout gear, a massage, or a healthy meal. Rewards provide positive reinforcement and make the process more enjoyable.
1. **Focus on the Positive:**
   - Instead of viewing exercise as a chore, focus on the positive aspects, such as how it makes you feel, the health benefits, and the progress you're making. Developing a positive mindset around exercise can help you look forward to your workouts.
1. **Visualize Your Success:**
   - Take a few moments each day to visualize yourself achieving your fitness goals. Whether it's lifting a heavier weight, crossing the finish line of a race, or simply feeling healthier, visualization can reinforce your commitment and boost motivation.

By incorporating these strategies into your routine, you'll build a sustainable workout habit that becomes a natural part of your daily life.

Overcoming Plateaus

Fitness plateaus are a common challenge, where progress stalls despite consistent effort. Overcoming these plateaus requires strategic adjustments to your workout routine and mindset:

1. **Vary Your Workouts:**
   - If you've been doing the same exercises for weeks or months, your body may have adapted, leading to a plateau. Introduce new exercises, change the order of your routine, or try different types of workouts to shock your muscles and reignite progress.
1. **Increase Intensity:**
   - Boost the intensity of your workouts by adding more weight, increasing the number of sets or reps, or reducing rest time between exercises. High-Intensity Interval Training (HIIT) is another effective way to break through plateaus by challenging your body with intense bursts of activity.
1. **Focus on Weak Points:**
   - Identify areas where you might be weaker or less developed and focus on strengthening them. For example, if you've hit a plateau in your upper body strength, incorporate more targeted exercises for your shoulders, back, or arms.
1. **Adjust Your Diet:**
   -

Nutrition plays a critical role in fitness progress. If you've hit a plateau, consider reviewing your diet to ensure you're getting the right balance of macronutrients (protein, carbohydrates, fats) to support your goals. Sometimes, small changes in your diet can make a big difference in your performance and recovery.

1. **Get Adequate Rest:**
   - Overtraining can lead to plateaus and even regression in progress. Ensure you're giving your body enough time to recover between workouts. Incorporating rest days, getting quality sleep, and managing stress are all important for breaking through plateaus.

1. **Set New Goals:**
   - If you've reached a major goal, it's natural for motivation to wane. Set new, challenging goals to reignite your drive. These goals can be related to strength, endurance, flexibility, or even trying a new sport or activity.

1. **Reevaluate Your Plan:**
   - Sometimes, a plateau is a sign that your workout plan needs a refresh. Take a step back and reevaluate your routine, considering what's working and what might need to change. Consulting with a fitness coach or trainer can also provide new insights and strategies.

1. **Stay Positive:**
   -

Plateaus can be frustrating, but they're a normal part of the fitness journey. Stay positive and patient, recognizing that progress isn't always linear. Trust the process and stay committed to your long-term goals.

By implementing these strategies, you can overcome plateaus and continue making progress towards your fitness objectives.

Keeping Your Workouts Fun and Engaging

One of the best ways to stay motivated and consistent with your workouts is to keep them fun and engaging. Here's how to inject some excitement into your routine:

1. **Try New Activities:**
   - Don't be afraid to experiment with new types of exercise. Whether it's trying a dance class, joining a sports league, or taking up rock climbing, new activities can challenge your body in different ways and keep things interesting.
1. **Incorporate Music:**
   - Create a playlist of your favorite high-energy songs to power through your workouts. Music can be a powerful motivator, helping you push through tough exercises and enjoy the process more.
1. **Join a Fitness Community:**
   - Engage with a fitness community, whether online or in-person. Group classes, workout challenges, or fitness forums can provide a sense of camaraderie and make exercise more enjoyable.
1. **Set Up Mini-Challenges:**
   - Introduce mini-challenges into your routine to keep things exciting. For example, you might challenge yourself to do a certain number of push-ups in a minute, beat your previous running time, or try a new yoga pose each week.

1. **Use Fitness Apps or Gadgets:**
    - Fitness apps, wearables, and gadgets can make tracking your progress and achieving goals more fun. Many apps offer gamified experiences, virtual rewards, and social features that can add an extra layer of engagement to your workouts.
1. **Change Your Environment:**
    - Sometimes a change of scenery can make all the difference. Try working out in different locations, such as a park, the beach, or even a new room in your home. Fresh surroundings can re-energize your routine and make exercise feel less monotonous.
1. **Incorporate Play:**
    - Find ways to make your workouts more playful. For example, you might play a game of tag with your kids, have a dance-off, or incorporate agility drills that feel more like games than exercise. Adding an element of play can make workouts feel less like a chore and more like fun.
1. **Focus on the Mind-Body Connection:**
    - Practice mindfulness during your workouts by focusing on your breathing, muscle engagement, and how your body feels during each movement. This can deepen your connection to the exercise and make it more satisfying.

By keeping your workouts fun and engaging, you're more likely to stick with them over the long term, ensuring that you continue to make progress and enjoy the journey.

Staying motivated and consistent with your workouts is key to achieving your fitness goals. By building a strong workout habit, overcoming plateaus, and keeping your routines fun and engaging, you'll be well on your way to a healthier, stronger, and more fulfilled version of yourself.

Chapter 13: Nutrition Tips for Optimal Performance

Proper nutrition is a cornerstone of any successful fitness regimen. The foods you eat and the fluids you drink directly impact your energy levels, workout performance, recovery, and overall health. This chapter provides essential nutrition tips to fuel your workouts, explains the importance of hydration, and offers simple, healthy recipes to support your fitness goals.

Eating Right for Your Workouts

What you eat before, during, and after your workouts can significantly influence your performance and recovery. Here's how to optimize your nutrition to get the most out of your exercise routine:

1. **Pre-Workout Nutrition:**
   - **Carbohydrates:** Carbohydrates are your body's primary source of energy, especially during high-intensity workouts. Eating a meal or snack rich in complex carbohydrates 1-3 hours before your workout can help ensure you have the energy needed to perform at your best. Examples include whole-grain bread, oatmeal, brown rice, or sweet potatoes.
   - **Protein:** Including a moderate amount of protein in your pre-workout meal can help support muscle repair and growth. Opt for lean sources like chicken, turkey, eggs, or Greek yogurt.
   - **Healthy Fats:** While fats are a slower-burning fuel source, a small amount of healthy fats can help sustain energy levels during longer workouts. Avocados, nuts, seeds, and olive oil are good options.

○

Timing: Aim to eat a balanced meal 2-3 hours before your workout. If you're short on time, a small snack 30-60 minutes before exercise can also be effective, such as a banana with peanut butter or a protein smoothie.

1. **Intra-Workout Nutrition:**

   ○

   Hydration: Staying hydrated during your workout is crucial for maintaining performance and preventing fatigue. Water is typically sufficient for most workouts, but for sessions lasting longer than 60 minutes, or in hot and humid conditions, you may benefit from a sports drink that replenishes electrolytes.

   ○

   Carbohydrates: For endurance activities lasting longer than 90 minutes, consider consuming easily digestible carbohydrates like energy gels, fruit, or a sports drink to maintain blood glucose levels and delay fatigue.

1. **Post-Workout Nutrition:**

   ○

   Protein: Consuming protein after your workout is essential for muscle recovery and growth. Aim for 20-30 grams of high-quality protein within 30-60 minutes after exercise. Good sources include whey protein, lean meats, fish, eggs, or plant-based proteins like tofu or legumes.

   ○

   Carbohydrates: Replenishing glycogen stores with carbohydrates after your workout is important, especially if you have another training session within the next 24 hours. Pair your post-workout protein with a source of complex carbohydrates like brown rice, quinoa, or sweet potatoes.

   ○

Healthy Fats: While not as critical immediately post-workout, incorporating healthy fats into your recovery meals can help reduce inflammation and support overall health. Add a small amount of avocado, nuts, seeds, or olive oil to your post-workout meal.

-

Timing: The post-workout window is often referred to as the "anabolic window," where nutrient intake can maximize recovery. While it's important to refuel within 30-60 minutes after exercise, the total intake over the course of the day is equally important.

By strategically timing your meals and snacks around your workouts, you can optimize your energy levels, performance, and recovery, helping you reach your fitness goals more efficiently.

Hydration: The Key to Success

Hydration is a critical component of athletic performance and overall health. Proper hydration helps regulate body temperature, transport nutrients, lubricate joints, and eliminate waste. Here's how to stay hydrated and ensure you're drinking enough fluids to support your fitness routine:

1. **Daily Hydration Needs:**
   -
   The amount of water you need varies depending on factors like your age, gender, activity level, and climate. A general guideline is to drink at least 8-10 cups (2-2.5 liters) of water per day, but athletes and those engaging in intense exercise may need more.
1. **Pre-Workout Hydration:**
   -
   Start your workout well-hydrated by drinking 16-20 ounces (0.5-0.6 liters) of water 2-3 hours before

exercise. About 20-30 minutes before your workout, drink another 8 ounces (0.24 liters) of water.

1. **During Workout Hydration:**
   -

   Sip on water regularly throughout your workout, aiming for 7-10 ounces (0.2-0.3 liters) every 10-20 minutes. If your workout lasts longer than an hour, or if you're exercising in hot or humid conditions, consider a sports drink that provides electrolytes like sodium and potassium to help replace what you lose through sweat.

1. **Post-Workout Hydration:**
   -

   After your workout, rehydrate by drinking 16-24 ounces (0.5-0.7 liters) of water for every pound (0.45 kg) of body weight lost during exercise. Weighing yourself before and after a workout can help determine how much fluid you need to replace. Additionally, consuming a beverage with electrolytes can aid in rehydration, especially after intense or prolonged exercise.

1. **Signs of Dehydration:**
   -

   Pay attention to signs of dehydration, which can include thirst, dry mouth, dark urine, fatigue, dizziness, and headaches. If you notice these symptoms, increase your fluid intake immediately.

1. **Electrolytes:**
   -

   Electrolytes, including sodium, potassium, magnesium, and calcium, play a vital role in maintaining fluid balance and muscle function. If you're sweating heavily or exercising for long periods, consider replenishing electrolytes through sports drinks, coconut water, or electrolyte tablets.

By prioritizing hydration before, during, and after exercise, you can maintain optimal performance, reduce the risk of cramps and heat-related illnesses, and support overall well-being.

Simple, Healthy Recipes for Fitness Enthusiasts

Eating healthy doesn't have to be complicated. Here are some simple, nutritious recipes that are perfect for fueling your workouts and supporting recovery:

1. **Overnight Oats with Berries and Nuts**
   - **Ingredients:**
       1. 1/2 cup rolled oats
       2. 1/2 cup unsweetened almond milk (or your choice of milk)
       3. 1/4 cup Greek yogurt
       4. 1 tablespoon chia seeds
       5. 1/2 cup mixed berries (blueberries, strawberries, raspberries)
       6. 1 tablespoon chopped nuts (almonds, walnuts, or pecans)
       7. 1 teaspoon honey or maple syrup (optional)
   - **Instructions:**
       1. In a mason jar or bowl, combine oats, almond milk, Greek yogurt, and chia seeds. Stir well.
       2. Top with mixed berries and chopped nuts. Drizzle with honey or maple syrup if desired.
       3. Cover and refrigerate overnight.
       4. In the morning, give it a stir and enjoy a delicious, nutrient-packed breakfast.
1. **Grilled Chicken and Quinoa Salad**

o

Ingredients:

1. 1 cup cooked quinoa
2. 1 grilled chicken breast, sliced
3. 1 cup mixed greens (spinach, arugula, kale)
4. 1/2 cup cherry tomatoes, halved
5. 1/4 cup cucumber, sliced
6. 1/4 avocado, sliced
7. 1 tablespoon olive oil
8. 1 tablespoon lemon juice
9. Salt and pepper to taste

o

Instructions:

1. In a large bowl, combine cooked quinoa, mixed greens, cherry tomatoes, cucumber, and avocado.
2. Top with sliced grilled chicken breast.
3. Drizzle with olive oil and lemon juice. Season with salt and pepper to taste.
4. Toss gently to combine and serve.

1. **Protein-Packed Smoothie**

   o

Ingredients:

1. 1 scoop protein powder (whey, plant-based, or your choice)
2. 1 banana
3. 1/2 cup frozen berries
4. 1 tablespoon almond butter
5. 1 cup unsweetened almond milk (or your choice of milk)
6. 1 handful spinach (optional)
7. 1 teaspoon honey or maple syrup (optional)

o

Instructions:

1. Add all ingredients to a blender.
2. Blend until smooth and creamy.
3. Pour into a glass and enjoy as a quick post-workout meal or snack.

1. **Sweet Potato and Black Bean Tacos**
   -

Ingredients:

1. 1 large sweet potato, peeled and cubed
2. 1 can black beans, drained and rinsed
3. 1 tablespoon olive oil
4. 1/2 teaspoon cumin
5. 1/2 teaspoon smoked paprika
6. Salt and pepper to taste
7. Small corn or whole wheat tortillas
8. Toppings: avocado slices, salsa, chopped cilantro, lime wedges

   -

Instructions:

1. Preheat oven to 400°F (200°C).
2. Toss cubed sweet potatoes with olive oil, cumin, smoked paprika, salt, and pepper. Spread on a baking sheet.
3. Roast for 25-30 minutes, until tender and slightly crispy.
4. Warm tortillas and fill with roasted sweet potatoes and black beans.
5. Add desired toppings, such as avocado, salsa, cilantro, and a squeeze of lime.
6. Serve immediately and enjoy a delicious, plant-based meal.

1. **Baked Salmon with Steamed Vegetables**
   -

Ingredients:

1. 2 salmon fillets
2. 1 tablespoon olive oil
3. 1 tablespoon lemon juice
4. 1 teaspoon garlic powder
5. Salt and pepper to taste
6. Mixed vegetables (broccoli, carrots, green beans) for steaming

o

Instructions:

1. Preheat oven to 375°F (190°C).
2. Place salmon fillets on a baking sheet. Drizzle with olive oil and lemon juice. Sprinkle with garlic powder, salt, and pepper.
3. Bake for 12-15 minutes, until salmon is cooked through and flakes easily with a fork.
4. While the salmon is baking, steam mixed vegetables until tender.
5. Serve the baked salmon with steamed vegetables for a nutrient-rich, balanced meal.

These simple, healthy recipes are designed to support your fitness goals by providing balanced nutrition that fuels your workouts, aids in recovery, and keeps you energized throughout the day.

Optimal nutrition is essential for achieving peak performance in your workouts and maintaining overall health. By eating the right foods at the right times, staying hydrated, and incorporating nutritious recipes into your diet, you'll be well-equipped to reach your fitness goals and enjoy a healthier, more vibrant lifestyle.

Chapter 14: Safety and Injury Prevention

Safety and injury prevention are crucial aspects of any fitness routine. Whether you're a beginner or an experienced athlete, understanding how to exercise safely and recognizing the signs of potential injuries can help you avoid setbacks and keep your fitness journey on track. This chapter will cover common workout injuries, provide tips for safe exercise at home, and discuss the importance of rest and recovery.

Recognizing Common Workout Injuries

Understanding the most common workout injuries and their symptoms can help you identify issues early and take action to prevent them from worsening. Here are some of the most frequent injuries associated with exercise:

1. **Strains and Sprains:**
   - **Description:** Strains occur when a muscle or tendon (which connects muscle to bone) is overstretched or torn. Sprains involve the overstretching or tearing of ligaments (which connect bones to each other).
   - **Common Causes:** Strains and sprains often result from improper warm-up, overuse, sudden movements, or lifting weights that are too heavy.
   - **Symptoms:** Pain, swelling, bruising, and limited range of motion in the affected area.
1. **Tendonitis:**
   - **Description:** Tendonitis is inflammation of a tendon, typically caused by repetitive stress or overuse.
   -

Common Causes: Activities that involve repetitive motions, such as running, swimming, or lifting weights, can lead to tendonitis, particularly in areas like the shoulders, elbows, and knees.

o

Symptoms: Pain, tenderness, and mild swelling near the affected tendon, especially during movement.

1. **Runner's Knee (Patellofemoral Pain Syndrome):**

   o

   Description: Runner's knee is a common overuse injury that causes pain around the kneecap.

   o

   Common Causes: Running, jumping, and other high-impact activities, especially when performed with improper form or on hard surfaces.

   o

   Symptoms: Pain around or behind the kneecap, particularly when walking down stairs, squatting, or sitting for long periods.

1. **Shin Splints (Medial Tibial Stress Syndrome):**

   o

   Description: Shin splints refer to pain along the inner edge of the shinbone (tibia), often due to overuse or improper footwear.

   o

   Common Causes: Running on hard surfaces, wearing unsupportive shoes, and increasing workout intensity too quickly.

   o

   Symptoms: Sharp or throbbing pain along the shin, especially during or after physical activity.

1. **Lower Back Pain:**

   o

   Description: Lower back pain can result from muscle strain, poor posture, or improper lifting technique.

○

Common Causes: Lifting heavy weights with poor form, sudden twisting movements, and prolonged periods of sitting or standing without proper support.

○

Symptoms: Dull or sharp pain in the lower back, stiffness, and difficulty bending or twisting.

1. **Rotator Cuff Injuries:**

    ○

    Description: The rotator cuff is a group of muscles and tendons that stabilize the shoulder. Injuries to the rotator cuff can range from inflammation to tears.

    ○

    Common Causes: Repetitive overhead motions, lifting weights with improper form, and falls or sudden impacts.

    ○

    Symptoms: Shoulder pain, weakness, and limited range of motion, especially during overhead activities.

Recognizing the early signs of these injuries and addressing them promptly can prevent more serious issues. If you experience persistent pain, swelling, or discomfort that doesn't improve with rest, it's important to seek medical advice.

Tips for Safe Exercise at Home

Exercising at home offers convenience and flexibility, but it's important to prioritize safety to prevent injuries. Here are some tips for creating a safe workout environment and practicing safe exercise habits at home:

1. **Create a Safe Workout Space:**

    ○

Clear the Area: Ensure your workout space is free from clutter, furniture, and other obstacles that could cause you to trip or fall. If you're using equipment like weights or resistance bands, store them safely when not in use.

o

Choose a Non-Slip Surface: If possible, work out on a non-slip surface like a yoga mat or carpet. This helps prevent slips and provides cushioning for your joints.

o

Ensure Adequate Lighting: Make sure your workout area is well-lit so you can see clearly and avoid accidents.

1. **Warm Up Properly:**

   o

   Importance of Warming Up: A proper warm-up increases blood flow to your muscles, prepares your body for exercise, and reduces the risk of injury. Spend 5-10 minutes warming up with dynamic stretches, light cardio, or mobility exercises before jumping into your workout.

1. **Focus on Form and Technique:**

   o

   Importance of Proper Form: Using proper form is essential for preventing injuries, especially when performing strength training exercises. Take the time to learn correct techniques, and start with lighter weights or simpler movements before progressing to more advanced exercises.

   o

   Use Mirrors: If possible, use a mirror to check your form while exercising. This can help you make adjustments and ensure you're performing movements correctly.

1. **Listen to Your Body:**

   o

Avoid Overtraining: Pushing yourself too hard can lead to overtraining, fatigue, and injuries. Pay attention to your body's signals, and don't be afraid to take rest days or modify your workouts if you're feeling sore or tired.

- **Stop if You Feel Pain:** Discomfort and muscle fatigue are normal during exercise, but sharp pain is a warning sign. If you experience pain during a workout, stop immediately and assess the situation. Continuing to exercise through pain can exacerbate injuries.

1. **Stay Hydrated:**

   - **Importance of Hydration:** Dehydration can lead to muscle cramps, dizziness, and fatigue, increasing the risk of injury. Drink water before, during, and after your workout to stay hydrated and maintain optimal performance.

1. **Use Equipment Safely:**

   - **Check Your Equipment:** Regularly inspect your workout equipment, such as resistance bands, dumbbells, and exercise mats, for wear and tear. Using damaged equipment can lead to accidents and injuries.

   - **Follow Instructions:** If you're using new equipment or trying a new exercise, read the instructions or watch tutorials to ensure you're using it correctly.

1. **Cool Down and Stretch:**

   - **Importance of Cooling Down:** After your workout, take 5-10 minutes to cool down with gentle stretches and deep breathing. This helps your body return to its resting state, reduces muscle stiffness, and promotes flexibility.

By following these safety tips, you can reduce the risk of injuries and create a safe, effective workout environment at home.

When to Rest and Recover

Rest and recovery are essential components of any fitness routine. Giving your body time to recover between workouts allows your muscles to repair and grow, reduces the risk of overtraining, and improves overall performance. Here's how to incorporate rest and recovery into your fitness plan:

1. **Understand the Importance of Rest:**
   - **Muscle Repair and Growth:** When you exercise, particularly during strength training, you create small tears in your muscle fibers. Rest days allow your body to repair these tears, leading to muscle growth and increased strength.
   - **Preventing Overtraining:** Overtraining occurs when you don't allow enough time for recovery between workouts, leading to fatigue, decreased performance, and a higher risk of injury. Regular rest days help prevent overtraining and keep you feeling strong and energized.
1. **Schedule Regular Rest Days:**
   - **Frequency of Rest Days:** Aim to include at least one or two rest days per week, depending on your fitness level and the intensity of your workouts. On rest days, focus on light activities like walking, stretching, or yoga to keep your body moving without straining your muscles.
1. **Incorporate Active Recovery:**
   -

Benefits of Active Recovery: Active recovery involves low-intensity exercise that promotes blood flow and aids in muscle recovery. Activities like swimming, cycling, or gentle yoga can help reduce muscle soreness and improve flexibility without adding additional stress to your body.

1. **Prioritize Sleep:**
   - **Importance of Sleep:** Sleep is crucial for recovery, as it's during sleep that your body produces growth hormone and repairs muscle tissue. Aim for 7-9 hours of quality sleep per night to support your fitness goals and overall health.

1. **Listen to Your Body:**
   - **Recognize Signs of Overtraining:** If you notice symptoms like persistent fatigue, decreased performance, irritability, or increased susceptibility to illness, you may be overtraining. In these cases, it's important to take a break, reduce workout intensity, or adjust your training plan to include more rest.

1. **Use Recovery Techniques:**
   - **Stretching and Foam Rolling:** Incorporate stretching and foam rolling into your routine to release muscle tension, improve flexibility, and enhance recovery. Foam rolling helps break up muscle knots and increases blood flow to the muscles, promoting faster recovery.
   - **Cold Therapy:** Applying ice or cold packs to sore muscles can help reduce inflammation and speed up recovery. Cold baths or contrast baths (alternating between hot and cold water) are also effective recovery methods.
   -

Nutrition for Recovery: Fuel your recovery with a balanced diet that includes adequate protein, healthy fats, and carbohydrates. Nutrient-dense foods like fruits, vegetables, lean proteins, and whole grains provide the building blocks your body needs to repair and grow.

1. **Adjust Your Routine as Needed:**

   -
     Be Flexible: It's important to be flexible with your workout routine and adjust it based on how your body feels. If you're feeling unusually sore or tired, consider taking an extra rest day or swapping a high-intensity workout for a low-impact activity.

By incorporating regular rest and recovery into your fitness plan, you'll enhance your performance, reduce the risk of injury, and ensure long-term success in your fitness journey.

Prioritizing safety and injury prevention is key to maintaining a consistent and effective workout routine. By recognizing common workout injuries, practicing safe exercise habits, and understanding the importance of rest and recovery, you can protect your body, stay motivated, and continue making progress toward your fitness goals.

Conclusion

The Long-Term Benefits of Home Workouts

Home workouts offer a range of long-term benefits that extend far beyond physical fitness. They provide a convenient, cost-effective, and adaptable way to stay active and healthy, regardless of your lifestyle or schedule. By committing to a regular home workout routine, you can enjoy the following long-term advantages:

1. **Sustainability:**
   - Home workouts are incredibly sustainable. Without the need for a gym membership or travel time, it's easier to maintain a consistent fitness routine, even when life gets busy. This consistency is key to achieving and maintaining long-term fitness goals.
1. **Flexibility and Convenience:**
   - Working out at home allows you to exercise whenever it suits you, whether it's early in the morning, late at night, or during a lunch break. This flexibility makes it easier to fit fitness into your day, reducing the likelihood of missed workouts.
1. **Cost Savings:**
   - Home workouts eliminate the need for expensive gym memberships, personal trainers, and travel costs. With just a few pieces of basic equipment— or even just your bodyweight—you can achieve a full-body workout without breaking the bank.
1. **Customization:**
   - When you work out at home, you have complete control over your fitness routine. You can tailor your workouts to your specific goals, preferences,

and fitness level, ensuring that your exercise program is both effective and enjoyable.

1. **Privacy and Comfort:**
   - Exercising in the comfort of your own home provides a level of privacy that's often lacking in a gym environment. This can be particularly beneficial for those who are self-conscious or prefer to work out alone. You can focus entirely on your fitness journey without distractions or comparisons.
1. **Improved Mental Health:**
   - Regular exercise, including home workouts, is proven to reduce stress, anxiety, and depression. The mental health benefits of staying active at home contribute to a more balanced, fulfilling life.
1. **Long-Term Health Benefits:**
   - Consistent home workouts help you build and maintain muscle, improve cardiovascular health, enhance flexibility and mobility, and reduce the risk of chronic diseases such as obesity, heart disease, and diabetes. The long-term health benefits are profound, contributing to a higher quality of life as you age.

Staying Fit for Life Without the Gym

Staying fit for life doesn't require a gym membership or fancy equipment. By embracing the principles and practices outlined in this book, you can achieve and maintain a high level of fitness entirely from home. Here are some key strategies for sustaining your fitness journey over the long term:

1. **Make Fitness a Lifestyle:**
   -

Integrate physical activity into your daily life, not just as a task to be completed but as a habit that enhances your well-being. Whether it's a morning workout, an evening walk, or active hobbies, find ways to stay active that you enjoy and can stick with for the long haul.

1. **Set and Revisit Goals:**
   - Regularly set new fitness goals to keep yourself motivated and challenged. As you achieve your goals, celebrate your progress and set new ones to continue growing and improving. This ongoing process keeps your fitness journey dynamic and engaging.

1. **Embrace Variety:**
   - Keep your workouts fresh and exciting by incorporating a variety of exercises and routines. Try new activities, explore different workout styles, and challenge yourself with advanced techniques as you progress. Variety not only prevents boredom but also helps you achieve a well-rounded fitness level.

1. **Prioritize Balance:**
   - Strive for balance in your fitness routine by including strength training, cardio, flexibility, and mobility exercises. This balanced approach ensures that all aspects of your physical health are addressed, reducing the risk of injury and improving overall performance.

1. **Listen to Your Body:**
   - As you continue on your fitness journey, it's important to listen to your body and adjust your routine as needed. Rest when necessary, recover properly, and modify exercises to suit your current

fitness level and needs. This mindful approach helps you avoid burnout and sustain your fitness efforts over the long term.

1. **Stay Motivated and Consistent:**
   -

Maintaining motivation and consistency is key to long-term fitness success. Use the tips and strategies outlined in this book to stay motivated, overcome challenges, and keep your workouts engaging. Remember that consistency, even in small doses, is more important than perfection.

Final Words of Encouragement

Embarking on a home workout journey is a powerful step toward improving your health, fitness, and overall quality of life. By choosing to stay active and make fitness a priority, you're investing in yourself—both physically and mentally. Remember that fitness is not a destination but a lifelong journey. It's about progress, not perfection.

There will be days when motivation wanes or life gets in the way, but don't let temporary setbacks discourage you. Every effort, no matter how small, contributes to your long-term success. Celebrate your achievements, learn from your challenges, and keep moving forward.

You have the tools, knowledge, and determination to stay fit and healthy without ever needing to step foot in a gym. Trust in your ability to create and sustain a fitness routine that works for you, and enjoy the countless benefits that come with an active, healthy lifestyle.

Here's to your health, strength, and continued success—both now and for years to come. Keep pushing, keep striving, and most importantly, keep moving. You've got this!

Appendix

Recommended Fitness Apps and Resources

In the digital age, there are countless apps and online resources that can enhance your home workout experience, help you stay on track, and provide support and motivation. Here's a list of some of the most useful fitness apps and resources:

1. **MyFitnessPal**
   -
     Description: A comprehensive app for tracking your diet and exercise. MyFitnessPal allows you to log your meals, track your calorie intake, and monitor your macronutrient balance. It also features a large database of exercises and can sync with various fitness devices.
   -
     Platforms: iOS, Android, Web
1. **Fitbod**
   -
     Description: Fitbod creates personalized strength training plans based on your fitness level, goals, and available equipment. It adapts your workout plan as you progress, ensuring continuous improvement.
   -
     Platforms: iOS, Android
1. **Nike Training Club**
   -
     Description: Nike Training Club offers a variety of guided workouts, ranging from strength training and cardio to yoga and mobility. The app provides video demonstrations and expert tips, making it easy to follow along at home.
   -
     Platforms: iOS, Android

1. **Headspace**

    o

    Description: While not strictly a fitness app, Headspace is a popular meditation app that offers guided sessions to help reduce stress, improve focus, and enhance mental well-being—important aspects of a balanced fitness routine.

    o

    Platforms: iOS, Android, Web

1. **Strava**

    o

    Description: Ideal for runners and cyclists, Strava tracks your routes, pace, and distance, and allows you to connect with a community of athletes. The app also offers challenges and leaderboards to keep you motivated.

    o

    Platforms: iOS, Android, Web

1. **JEFIT**

    o

    Description: JEFIT is a workout planner and fitness tracker that offers pre-designed workout plans and the ability to create your own. The app tracks your progress, logs your workouts, and provides exercise tutorials.

    o

    Platforms: iOS, Android, Web

1. **Yoga with Adriene**

    o

    Description: A popular YouTube channel offering free yoga classes for all levels. Adriene's approachable and gentle teaching style makes it easy to incorporate yoga into your fitness routine, whether you're a beginner or experienced yogi.

    o

    Platforms: YouTube, Web

1. **Down Dog**

o

Description: Down Dog offers customizable yoga sessions that allow you to choose the style, length, and intensity of your practice. The app provides clear instructions and high-quality video demonstrations.

o

Platforms: iOS, Android, Web

1. **Peloton**

   o

   Description: Peloton offers a wide range of live and on-demand fitness classes, including cycling, running, strength training, yoga, and more. While Peloton is known for its bike and treadmill, the app can be used independently for other types of workouts.

   o

   Platforms: iOS, Android, Web

1. **Fitness Blender**

   o

   Description: Fitness Blender is a free online resource that offers a huge library of full-length workout videos, including HIIT, strength training, cardio, and flexibility routines. The website also features workout plans and fitness tips.

   o

   Platforms: YouTube, Web

These apps and resources can enhance your home workouts, provide structure and guidance, and keep you motivated on your fitness journey.

Workout Trackers and Journals

Tracking your workouts and progress is an essential part of staying consistent and achieving your fitness goals. Whether you prefer digital tools or traditional paper journals, here are some recommended options for tracking your fitness journey:

1. **Fitbit**
   - **Description:** Fitbit devices track your daily activity, including steps, distance, calories burned, and sleep patterns. The accompanying app allows you to log workouts, monitor your heart rate, and set fitness goals.
   - **Platforms:** iOS, Android, Web
1. **Strong**
   - **Description:** Strong is a popular app for tracking strength training workouts. It allows you to log sets, reps, and weights, and provides detailed insights into your progress over time.
   - **Platforms:** iOS, Android
1. **Pen and Paper Fitness Journal**
   - **Description:** A simple, traditional method for tracking your workouts. Use a dedicated fitness journal or notebook to log your exercises, sets, reps, and weights. This method allows for customization and personal reflection.
1. **Moleskine Wellness Journal**
   - **Description:** Moleskine's Wellness Journal is designed to help you track your fitness and wellness journey. It includes sections for logging workouts, tracking nutrition, setting goals, and reflecting on your progress.
   - **Platforms:** Physical journal
1. **BodyMinder Workout and Exercise Journal**

o

Description: The BodyMinder Workout and Exercise Journal is a physical logbook that allows you to track your workouts, including cardio, strength training, and flexibility exercises. It also includes space for notes on nutrition and goals.

o

Platforms: Physical journal

1. **Google Sheets or Excel**

   o

   Description: If you prefer a digital but customizable approach, using Google Sheets or Excel to create your own workout tracker can be an effective solution. You can design your tracker to include exercises, sets, reps, weights, and progress over time.

1. **Bullet Journal**

   o

   Description: A bullet journal is a customizable analog system that you can use to track your workouts, set fitness goals, and reflect on your progress. It's highly adaptable, allowing you to design your fitness tracking system in a way that suits your needs.

   o

   Platforms: Physical journal

Whether you choose an app, a physical journal, or a combination of both, tracking your workouts helps you stay accountable, recognize patterns, and celebrate your achievements.

Further Reading and Support

For those looking to deepen their understanding of fitness, nutrition, and overall well-being, here are some recommended books and resources:

1. **Books on Fitness and Exercise:**

    o

    "Starting Strength" by Mark Rippetoe: A comprehensive guide to strength training, focusing on fundamental lifts and proper technique. Ideal for beginners and intermediate lifters.

    o

    "The New Rules of Lifting" by Lou Schuler and Alwyn Cosgrove: A practical guide to strength training that includes detailed workout plans and insights into the science of lifting.

    o

    "You Are Your Own Gym" by Mark Lauren: A guide to bodyweight exercises that require no equipment, perfect for those who want to work out at home with minimal resources.

    o

    "Becoming a Supple Leopard" by Kelly Starrett: A book focused on mobility and movement, offering techniques to improve flexibility, prevent injury, and enhance performance.

1. **Books on Nutrition:**

    o

    "The Power of Habit" by Charles Duhigg: While not solely focused on fitness, this book explores the science of habits and how they can be applied to improve health and wellness.

    o

    "The Precision Nutrition System" by John Berardi and Ryan Andrews: A comprehensive guide to nutrition that provides practical advice and strategies for healthy eating, tailored to individual goals.

    o

"How Not to Die" by Michael Greger, M.D.: A book focused on plant-based nutrition and how diet can prevent and reverse common health conditions.

1. **Online Fitness Communities:**
   - **Reddit Fitness Communities:** Subreddits like r/Fitness, r/BodyweightFitness, and r/xxfitness (for women) offer advice, support, and motivation from a global community of fitness enthusiasts.
   - **Fitocracy:** An online fitness community and app that gamifies your fitness journey, allowing you to earn points and badges for completing workouts and achieving goals.
   - **MyFitnessPal Forums:** A community within the MyFitnessPal app where users can share tips, ask questions, and find support on their fitness and nutrition journey.
1. **Support from Professionals:**
   - **Personal Trainers:** If you're looking for personalized guidance, consider hiring a certified personal trainer who can create a custom workout plan and provide one-on-one coaching.
   - **Registered Dietitians:** For tailored nutrition advice, working with a registered dietitian can help you develop a diet plan that aligns with your fitness goals and health needs.
   - **Physical Therapists:** If you're dealing with injuries or want to prevent them, a physical therapist can provide exercises and strategies to help you stay healthy and active.

These books, resources, and communities can provide additional support, knowledge, and inspiration as you continue on your fitness journey.

The resources and tools provided in this appendix are designed to help you stay organized, motivated, and informed as you work towards your fitness goals. Whether you're tracking your workouts, exploring new apps, or diving into further reading, these recommendations will support you in maintaining a consistent and effective fitness routine.

www.ingramcontent.com/pod-product-compliance
Lightning Source LLC
Chambersburg PA
CBHW061354250726
48657CB00004B/1493